Adult Flatfoot

Guest Editor

STEVEN M. RAIKIN, MD

FOOT AND ANKLE CLINICS

www.foot.theclinics.com

Consulting Editor
MARK S. MYERSON, MD

June 2012 • Volume 17 • Number 2

SAUNDERS an imprint of ELSEVIER, Inc.

W.B. SAUNDERS COMPANY
A Division of Elsevier Inc.

1600 John F. Kennedy Blvd. • Suite 1800 • Philadelphia, PA 19103-2899

http://www.theclinics.com

FOOT AND ANKLE CLINICS Volume 17, Number 2
June 2012 ISSN 1083-7515, ISBN-13: 978-1-4557-3862-5

Editor: David Parsons
Developmental Editor: Teia Stone

Foot and Ankle Clinics (ISSN 1083-7515) is published quarterly by Elsevier, Inc., 360 Park Avenue South, New York, NY 10010-1710. Months of issue are March, June, September, and December. Periodicals postage paid at New York, NY, and additional mailing offices. Subscription price per year is $295.00 (US individuals), $386.00 (US institutions), $146.00 (US students), $336.00 (Canadian individuals), $456.00 (Canadian institutions), $201.00 (Canadian students), $433.00 (foreign individuals), $456.00 (foreign institutions), and $201.00 (foreign students). To receive student/resident rate, orders must be accompanied by name of affiliated institution, date of term, and the signature of program/residency coordinator on institution letterhead. Orders will be billed at individual rate until proof of status is received. Foreign air speed delivery is included in all *Clinics* subscription prices. All prices are subject to change without notice. **POSTMASTER:** Send address changes to *Foot and Ankle Clinics,* Elsevier Health Sciences Division, Subscription Customer Service, 3251 Riverport Lane, Maryland Heights, MO 63043. **Customer Service: 1-800-654-2452 (US and Canada). From outside of the United States and Canada, call 314-447-8871. Fax: 314-447-8029. E-mail: JournalsCustomerService-usa@elsevier.com (for print support); JournalsOnlineSupport-usa@elsevier.com (for online support).**

Reprints. For copies of 100 or more, of articles in this publication, please contact the Commercial Reprints Department, Elsevier Inc., 360 Park Avenue South, New York, NY 10010-1710. Tel.: 212-633-3812; Fax: 212-462-1935; E-mail: reprints@elsevier.com.

Printed and bound by CPI Group (UK) Ltd, Croydon, CR0 4YY

Transferred to Digital Print 2012

Contributors

CONSULTING EDITOR

MARK S. MYERSON, MD
Director, Institute for Foot and Ankle Reconstruction at Mercy, Mercy Medical Center, Baltimore, Maryland

GUEST EDITOR

STEVEN M. RAIKIN, MD
Director, Foot and Ankle Service; Professor, Orthopaedic Surgery, Rothman Institute and Thomas Jefferson University Hospital, Philadelphia, Pennsylvania

AUTHORS

JAMAL AHMAD, MD
Assistant Professor of Orthopaedic Surgery, Rothman Institute Orthopaedics at Thomas Jefferson University Hospital, Philadelphia, Pennsylvania

FERNANDO ÁLVAREZ, MD
Head, Foot and Ankle Unit, Orthopaedic Surgery Department, Hospital San Rafael, Barcelona, Spain

JOSEFINA ALVAREZ, MD
Orthopaedic Surgeon, Foot and Ankle Surgery Service, British Hospital, Montevideo, Uruguay

JOHN G. ANDERSON, MD
Orthopaedic Associates of Michigan, PC; Chairman, Department of Orthopaedic Surgery, Spectrum Health; Professor, Department of Orthopaedic Surgery, Michigan State University College of Human Medicine; Assistant Program Director, GRMEP Orthopaedic Surgery Residency Program; Co-Director, Grand Rapids Orthopaedic Foot and Ankle Fellowship, Grand Rapids, Michigan

MICHAEL S. ARONOW, MD
Associate Professor, Department of Orthopaedic Surgery, University of Connecticut School of Medicine, Farmington, Connecticut

GUSTAVO BACCA, MD
Fellow, Foot and Ankle Unit, Orthopaedic Surgery Department, Hospital San Rafael, Barcelona, Spain

ERIC M. BLUMAN, MD, PhD
Department of Orthopaedic Surgery, Brigham Foot and Ankle Center at the Faulkner, Brigham and Women's Hospital, Boston, Massachusetts

DONALD R. BOHAY, MD, FACS
Orthopaedic Associates of Michigan, PC; Associate Professor, Department of Orthopaedic Surgery, Michigan State University College of Human Medicine; Director, Grand Rapids Orthopaedic Foot and Ankle Fellowship, Grand Rapids, Michigan

JAMES D.F. CALDER, MD, FRCS (Tr & Orth)
Consultant Orthopaedic Surgeon, Department of Trauma and Orthopaedic Surgery, Chelsea and Westminster Hospital NHS Foundation Trust, London, United Kingdom

JOSEPH N. DANIEL, DO
Rothman Institute of Orthopaedics at Thomas Jefferson University Hospital, Philadelphia, Pennsylvania

PABLO FERNÁNDEZ DE RETANA, MD
Head, Orthopaedic Surgery Department, Hospital San Rafael, Barcelona, Spain

CHRISTOPHER E. GENTCHOS, MD
Foot & Ankle Orthopaedic Specialist, Concord Orthopaedics PA, Concord, New Hampshire

ABHIJIT R. GUHA, MBBS(Hons), MS(Orth), FRCS(Ed), FRCS(Tr & Orth)
Specialist Orthopaedic Registrar, Department of Trauma and Orthopaedics, University Hospital of Wales, Heath Park, Cardiff, Wales, United Kingdom

SAFET O. HATIC II, DO
Orthopedic Associates of SW Ohio, Dayton, Ohio

JEFFREY E. JOHNSON, MD
Professor, Department of Orthopedic Surgery; Chief, Foot and Ankle Service, Barnes-Jewish Hospital and Washington University School of Medicine, St Louis, Missouri

ALICIA LASALLE, MD
Orthopaedic Surgeon, Foot and Ankle Surgery Service, Police Hospital, Montevideo, Uruguay

JEREMY J. MCCORMICK, MD
Assistant Professor, Department of Orthopedic Surgery, Foot and Ankle Service, Barnes-Jewish Hospital and Washington University School of Medicine, St Louis, Missouri

U. ALFIERI MONTRASIO, MD
CTS Foot and Ankle, IRCCS Galeazzi, Milan, Italy

DAVID PEDOWITZ, MS, MD
Assistant Professor of Orthopaedic Surgery, Rothman Institute Orthopaedics at Thomas Jefferson University Hospital, Philadelphia, Pennsylvania

ANTHONY M. PERERA, MBChB, MRCS, MFSEM, PGDip (Med Law), FRCS (Orth)
Consultant Orthopaedic Surgeon, Department of Trauma and Orthopaedics, University Hospital of Wales, Heath Park, Cardiff, Wales, United Kingdom

TERRENCE M. PHILBIN, DO, FAOAO
Director, Foot and Ankle Service, Doctors Hospital Residency, Columbus; Orthopedic Foot and Ankle Center, Westerville, Ohio

STEVEN M. RAIKIN, MD
Director, Foot and Ankle Service; Professor, Orthopaedic Surgery, Rothman Institute of Orthopaedics at Thomas Jefferson University Hospital, Philadelphia, Pennsylvania

ANDREW J. ROCHE, FRCS (Tr & Orth)
Fellow in Foot and Ankle Surgery, Department of Trauma and Orthopaedic Surgery, Chelsea and Westminster Hospital NHS Foundation Trust, London, United Kingdom

V. JAMES SAMMARCO, MD
Cincinnati Sports Medicine & Orthopaedic Center, Cincinnati, Ohio

NURI SCHINCA, MD
Orthopaedic Surgeon, Foot and Ankle Surgery Service, British Hospital, Montevideo, Uruguay

JEREMY T. SMITH, MD
Department of Orthopaedic Surgery, Brigham Foot and Ankle Center at the Faulkner, Brigham and Women's Hospital, Boston, Massachusetts

ROSS TAYLOR, MD
Coastal Orthopedics, Conway, South Carolina

STEVEN W. THORPE, MD
Resident, Department of Orthopaedic Surgery, University of Pittsburgh Medical Center, Pittsburgh, Pennsylvania

F.G. USUELLI, MD
CTS Foot and Ankle, IRCCS Galeazzi, Milan, Italy

BRIAN S. WINTERS, MD
Resident, Orthopaedic Surgery, Rothman Institute of Othopaedics at Thomas Jefferson University Hospital, Philadelphia, Pennsylvania

DANE K. WUKICH, MD
Associate Professor of Orthopaedic Surgery and Chief, Foot and Ankle Division, Department of Orthopaedic Surgery, University of Pittsburgh Medical Center, Pittsburgh, Pennsylvania

Contents

Adult-acquired flatfoot occurs secondary to collapse of the medial longitudinal arch and can affect the rearfoot, ankle, and midfoot in different ways. Most current classification systems are based on a linear deformity progression as the pathologic condition worsens. Clinical experience, however, dictates that the deformity does not progress along a predictable path, and as such each level should be addressed and treated independently. The authors propose a classification scheme wherein the rearfoot (R), ankle (A), and midfoot (M) deformities are independently described and assessed, and they propose a systematic treatment approach to the adult-acquired flatfoot.

Flexible flatfoot is one of the most common deformities of the body. Arthroereisis procedures are designed to correct this deformity. Among them, the calcaneo-stop procedure, designed for pediatric treatment, has both biomechanical and proprioceptive properties. Results are reported similar to endorthesis procedure. The arthroereisis procedure can theoretically be applied to adults if combined with other procedures to obtain a stable plantigrade foot, but medium-term follow up studies are missing.

There is a paucity of information on adult coalitions without large, well-designed outcome studies. Current recommendations are thus similar to those for adolescents. Current recommendations include an initial trial of adequate nonoperative treatment in symptomatic coalitions. Unlike adolescent coalitions, nonoperative treatment may be even more effective in the adult patient as many are asymptomatic or discovered after injury. If nonoperative treatment fails, then surgical intervention is considered and tailored to the location of the coalition, existing advanced arthrosis, and any existing deformity. Similar to the adolescent, surgical treatment for adult calcaneonavicular coalitions typically involves an attempt at resection with some type of interposition.

> Acquired adult flatfoot is a challenging problem for orthopedic surgeons. Subtalar arthroereisis is a treatment option for stage IIA posterior tibial tendon dysfunction, as an alternative to calcaneal medializing osteotomy. In this article, the authors discuss the indications, surgical technique, results, and complications of subtalar arthroereisis in adult acquired flatfoot.

> Adult acquired flatfoot deformity (AAFD) is a complex problem with a wide variety of treatment options. No single procedure or group of procedures can be applied to all patients with AAFD. Careful physical examination and review of weight-bearing radiographs determines which patients have an associated forefoot varus deformity that may require correction at the time of flatfoot reconstruction. The choice of medial cuneiform osteotomy versus medial column fusion for correction of forefoot varus depends on the location and magnitude of the deformity, pressure of osteoarthritis and flexability of the medial column.

> Recurrence of deformity following soft tissue reconstruction, including tendon transfer, in the context of treatment for stage II flatfoot deformity represents a challenging problem for even the most experienced foot and ankle surgeon. The goals of treatment in flexible flatfoot should include restoration of alignment and alleviation of pain while minimizing stiffness, maintaining motion, and avoiding overcorrection. Arthrodesis should be reserved for fixed deformities or flexible deformities failing soft tissue reconstruction, including tendon transfer, where revision with extra-articular procedures is unlikely to facilitate adequate realignment and resolution of symptoms.

> Traditional surgical treatment for adults with a rigid, arthritic flatfoot is dual-incision triple arthrodesis, which has proved reliable and reproducible. Early complications include lateral wound problems, malunion, and nonunion. Long-term follow-up has shown adjacent joint arthritis at the ankle or midfoot. Although indications and surgical techniques have evolved and improved, it should be regarded as a salvage procedure. It

requires preoperative planning, meticulous preparation of bony surfaces, cognizance of hindfoot positioning, and rigidity of fixation, as well as enough experience on the part of the operating surgeon to anticipate postoperative problems and provide modifications in traditional technique.

Every alternative to triple arthrodesis in the rigid acquired flatfoot deformity is predicated on limiting the patient exposure to the complication associated with triple arthrodesis. When possible, avoiding arthrodesis of either the talonavicular and calcaneocuboid joints, with their higher nonunion rates, seems a cogent option. Successful treatment is dependent on thoughtful patient evaluation and examination, meticulous joint preparation, careful positioning with rigid fixation, and judicious use of adjunctive procedures to achieve the goal of a plantigrade foot that functions well and is minimally painful.

The authors discuss alternatives to fusion surgery for the treatment of rigid flatfoot deformity. Individual components of rigid flatfoot deformity are reviewed. Arthrodesis may be the only appropriate surgical procedure for some patients. In patients with limited arthritis, deformity correction and pain relief can be accomplished with a more limited fusion combined with corrective osteotomy and soft-tissue procedures. Triple arthrodesis and pan-talar arthrodesis can be avoided when only truly arthritic joints are fused and the correction of associated deformities such as equinus contracture, ankle and hindfoot valgus, midfoot abduction, and forefoot varus are done with the goal of joint preservation.

Dysfunction of the posterior tibial tendon leads to acquired adult flatfoot deformity (AAFD), which can be painful and disabling. The four stages of AAFD correlate to increasing deformity. Stage IV AAFD occurs when the talus tilts into valgus within the ankle mortise. Patients with a flexible deformity without advanced tibiotalar arthritis (stage IV-A) can be considered for a joint-sparing procedure. Patients with rigid valgus ankle deformity or flexible deformity accompanied by advanced tibiotalar arthritis (stage IV-B) should be considered for a joint-sacrificing procedure. The most reliable results for stage IV-B have been reported with tibiotalocalcaneal or pantalar arthrodesis.

FOOT AND ANKLE CLINICS

Preface

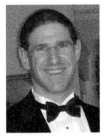

Steven M. Raikin, MD
Guest Editor

The understanding of the pathomechanics of the Adult Acquired Flatfoot (AAFF) has undergone a major evolution since its first description by Kulowski in 1936. Initially described purely as a disorder of the posterior tibial tendon, we now understand that the deformity additionally involves, among other contributors, the support of the spring ligament (which makes up part of the medial ligamentous support of the ankle) and as such the deltoid ligament, as well as a contribution from the midfoot through ligamentous laxity or degenerative collapse.

Along with this understanding has come an evolution in the classification and staging system from a simple three-part descriptor of the degree and rigidity of the deformity, to an ever more detailed description of the components of the deformity and how each of these influence management, both surgically and nonsurgically.

In constructing this edition of Foot and Ankle Clinics on the AAFF, I have compiled a team of experts from around the world to share their unique experience and knowledge in managing this complex condition. These surgeons from the United States, England, Italy, Spain, Uruguay, and Wales have generously shared their exceptional ability and time to enlighten us in differing ways to approach and manage these complex deformities. Their insights will significantly enhance the readers understanding of and capacity to treat patients with AAFF disorders.

I thank each of the contributors for the tremendous time and effort they have put into preparing their articles for this edition, as well as their spouses and children, who sacrificed their precious time with the authors to allow our education to be furthered.

Finally, thank you to Mark Myerson, MD, and the Elsevier staff for all the support and assistance in putting this edition together. It is the collaboration of all of these people that allows us to learn more, sharpen our abilities, and ultimately improve the lives and functioning of our patients.

Steven M. Raikin, MD
Rothman Institute of Orthopaedics at
Thomas Jefferson University Hospital
925 Chestnut Street
Philadelphia, PA 19107, USA

E-mail address:
steven.raikin@rothmaninstitute.com

Foot Ankle Clin N Am 17 (2012) xiii–xiii
doi:10.1016/j.fcl.2012.03.012

foot.theclinics.com

The RAM Classification
A Novel, Systematic Approach to the Adult-Acquired Flatfoot

Steven M. Raikin, MD*, Brian S. Winters, MD, Joseph N. Daniel, DO

KEYWORDS

- Flatfoot • Planovalgus • Classification • Posterior tibial tendon

KEY POINTS

- Adult-acquired flatfoot (AAFF) can develop from or result in deformities at the rearfoot (R), ankle (A), or midfoot (M).
- AAFF involving the rearfoot (R) should be classified and managed according to established criteria for posterior tibial tendon dysfunction.
- Not all ankle involvement (A) in AAFF is the same. Each patient ankle needs to be assessed individually and treatment tailored to the specific pattern of deformity.
- Midfoot involvement in AAFF can be secondary to rearfoot disease (posterior tibial tendon dysfunction) or the primary cause of the planovalgus. Involvement of this level needs to be carefully assessed clinically and radiographically and treatment tailored to the midfoot pattern of involvement in each foot.

The adult-acquired flatfoot (AAFF) is most commonly associated with dysfunction of the posterior tibial tendon (PTT) and presents clinically as a painful pes planus deformity.[1-5] From the time posterior tibial tendonitis was initially described in 1936 by Kulowski until 1983, little can be found throughout the literature pertaining to this topic aside from a few case series.[1,4] In 1983, Johnson was the first to discuss the signs and symptoms that resulted from rupture of the PTT.[4] He described a valgus deformity of the hindfoot and abduction deformity of the forefoot, which has since become the hallmark of this disorder.[1,3-6] From this work, he established the "too many toes" sign and the inability to perform a single-leg heel rise as indicators of loss of PTT function.[1,4-6]

In 1989, Johnson and Strom described a series of stages associated with dysfunction of the PTT and devised a useful classification system. Their system is based on the condition of the tendon, the position of the hindfoot, and flexibility

Rothman Institute of Orthopaedics at Thomas Jefferson University Hospital, 925 Chestnut Street, Philadelphia, PA 19107, USA
* Corresponding author.
E-mail address: steven.raikin@rothmaninstitute.com

Foot Ankle Clin N Am 17 (2012) 169–181
doi:10.1016/j.fcl.2012.03.002
1083-7515/12/$ – see front matter © 2012 Elsevier Inc. All rights reserved.

foot.theclinics.com

of the deformity.[1,3,6] The diagnosis and treatment of PTT dysfunction today has been organized around this staging scheme. The presentation of PTT dysfunction can range from tenosynovitis to a fixed pes planovalgus deformity with degenerative arthrosis and instability.[1-3,5-9] These changes follow a progressive course according to Johnson and Strom's initial classification system.[1,3,5,6] Stage 1 disease includes those patients who have tenderness, fullness, and tenosynovitis (with or without tendinopathy) without deformity. In stage 2 disease, patients have a dynamic, or flexible, deformity with some degree of hindfoot valgus malalignment, loss of the medial longitudinal arch, forefoot abduction, and forefoot varus. This stage has developed the most controversy in regard to treatment recommendations because of the tremendous variation in the anatomy, configuration, and location of the deformity and the many satisfactory operations that are available for correction.[3,9-11] Stage 3 disease is characterized by a fixed hindfoot valgus deformity, often accompanied by a fixed compensatory forefoot varus, which occurs to maintain a plantigrade foot. Johnson's classification system was subsequently modified by Myerson[12] with the addition of a fourth stage.[2,6,9,12] This more advanced stage described the involvement of the ankle joint and deltoid ligament.

Over the years, the understanding of the biomechanics of the arch and development of the flatfoot (currently termed the *adult-acquired flatfoot* because of the various causes in addition the PTT dysfunction) has evolved. Numerous investigators have since proposed variations of Johnson and Strom's system in an effort to encompass the expanded spectrum of AAFF and its associated deformities.[2,3,5-11] All continue to maintain their system's overall structure (stage 1–4) and the PTTs central role in the development of the deformity but have added new subclassifications.[2,3,6-9,11]

These alternate, more comprehensive systems increasingly acknowledge the involvement of the midfoot in the development of the AAFF, while noting the progressive effect of a dysfunctional PTT on the rearfoot and subsequently the ankle. They do not, however, account for the fact that deformity progression is not necessarily a linear process and may affect different zones around the foot and ankle (rearfoot, ankle, and midfoot) in various ways and degrees in different patients. Because of this lack, not every AAFF presents with a pattern that is consistent with the current classification systems. This inconsistency can serve as a source of confusion when trying to assign a specific patient to a certain grade or stage and in ultimately devising a treatment plan.

An ideal classification system not only needs to provide a reproducible description, but should also be easily applied to direct treatment and predict prognosis. Accordingly, the authors present a new classification for the AAFF wherein each level of deformity is assessed and graded independently of each other, both clinically and radiographically. This specificity allows the treating physician to classify and subsequently address each component of the deformity within a treatment algorithm and guide them in providing specific nonsurgical and surgical care.

RAM CLASSIFICATION

The RAM classification breaks the AAFF deformity into the individual components involved in the disease process (**Table 1**). The authors have maintained the grade I–III system and (a) and (b) subclassification currently in use but have applied these separately to the rearfoot (R), ankle (A), and midfoot (M).

Table 1
The RAM classification

	Rearfoot	Ankle	Midfoot
Ia	Tenosynovitis of PTT	Neutral alignment	Neutral alignment
Ib	PTT tendonitis without deformity	Mild valgus (<5°)	Mild flexible midfoot supination
IIa	Flexible planovalgus (<40% talar uncoverage, <30° Meary angle, incongruency angle 20° to 45°)	Valgus with deltoid insufficiency (no arthritis)	Midfoot supination without radiographic instability
IIb	Flexible planovalgus (>40% talar uncoverage, >30° Meary angle, incongruency angle >45°)	Valgus with deltoid insufficiency with tibiotalar arthritis	Midfoot supination with midfoot instability—no arthritis
IIIa	Fixed/arthritic planovalgus (<40% talar uncoverage, <30° Meary angle, incongruency angle 20° to 45°)	Valgus secondary to bone loss in the lateral tibial plafond (deltoid normal)	Arthritic changes isolated to medial column (navicular-medial cuneiform or first TMT joints)
IIIb	Fixed/arthritic planovalgus (>40% talar uncoverage, >30° Meary angle, incongruency angle >45°) —not correctable through triple arthrodesis	Valgus secondary to bone loss in the lateral tibial plafond and with deltoid insufficiency	Medial and middle column midfoot arthritic changes (usually with supination and/or abduction of the midfoot)

REARFOOT
Stage R-I

In stage I rearfoot disease, the patient presents with pain and often swelling over the PTT. Clinical examination reveals tenderness on direct palpation over the tendon, with pain exacerbated by resisted inversion and plantarflexion of the ankle. The arch alignment is well-maintained, and patients can usually perform a single-leg heel rise maneuver, albeit with pain. Young active patients and those with systemic inflammatory conditions such as rheumatoid arthritis are frequently affected, but older patients may present in early stages of the disease with these findings.

Stage R-Ia: tenosynovitis
In stage R-Ia tenosynovitis patients, the tendon itself is normal morphologically and functionally. The tenosynovium around the tendon is inflamed, resulting in pain. Radiographs are normal in these patients, whereas magnetic resonance imaging or ultrasound evaluation will reveal an intact PTT with normal structural integrity and signal. The surrounding tenosynovium is inflamed around the tendon.

Nonsurgical treatment is usually successful in this stage. This treatment includes temporary immobilization and antiinflammatory medication. If unsuccessful, a surgical tenosynovectomy is performed without surgery directly on the tendon. Medial rearfoot posted orthotic inserts should be used after successful treatment to minimize stress on the PTT. Recalcitrant stage R-Ia is most frequently seen in the presence of an inflammatory arthropathy.

Stage R-Ib: tendonitis/tendinosis

Patients with stage R-Ib tendonitis/tendinosis have structural damage to the PTT, either tendonitis or intrasubstance tearing. The tendon itself is weakened but remains intact and maintains its length, and the integrity of secondary arch support is not compromised. As such no deformity develops.

Nonsurgical treatment is usually successful in this stage. This treatment includes temporary immobilization and antiinflammatory medication. Once the tendonitis has resolved, a structured PTT-optimizing physical therapy program should be instituted and medial hindfoot posted orthotic inserts used. If unsuccessful, a molded ankle foot orthosis can be used for long-term control.

If nonsurgical management fails, surgery would include a débridement and repair of the PTT as necessary, combined with an augmenting tendon transfer procedure, usually with the flexor digitorum longus (FDL) tendon. There is no indication for an isolated PTT tendon repair without augmentation, unless the tear is due to an acute traumatic laceration.

Stage R-II

In stage II disease, the integrity of the PTT deteriorates and the tendon lengthens. This condition can occur as a result of progressive longitudinal tearing of the tendon or mucinous degeneration (tendinosis), with morphologic changes within the tendon itself, and can lead to rupture. Rupture does not, however, need to be present as suggested in prior classification systems.[2,3] As a result of tendon elongation, the arch of the midfoot starts to collapse. This occurrence can be seen clinically (hindfoot valgus, "too many toes" sign, decreased arch height), and radiographically (apex plantar collapse of Meary's talo–first metatarsal angle, uncoverage of the talar head at the talonavicular joint, talonavicular incongruency angle[13]). Patients will have increased difficulty with single-leg heel raise clinically. Whereas they can often perform this maneuver, they will not be able to do so repeatedly. While performing a double-limbed heel raise, the involved hindfoot will usually not be pulled into the normal degree of varus as seen on the unaffected side. The deformity is flexible and passively correctable in this stage. No arthritic changes are seen radiographically or on tertiary studies. Determining which substage of stage II the patient has is dependent on the amount of deformity present, particularly radiographically. As the deformity progresses and the spring ligament becomes increasingly incompetent, the talar head becomes less congruent within the talonavicular joint (seen as a more vertical and adducted talus) and the forefoot becomes more abducted. No absolute numbers exist to differentiate the two stages, but the authors propose ranges based on the literature. One should keep in mind when assessing these radiographs that the deformity is three-dimensional and some overlap between stages is not uncommon. Nonsurgical treatment follows the same protocol described in type R-Ib.

Stage R-IIa: mild to moderate deformity

Lateral weightbearing radiographs are assessed for the talo–first metatarsal alignment, or Meary's angle. In the AAFF, the angle is always apex plantar, with a normal angle of less than 4°. In stage IIa, the Meary's angle is between 4° and 30°. On the weightbearing anteroposterior (AP) radiographs, the uncoverage percentage at the talonavicular joint is between 20% and 40% and the incongruency angle is between 20° and 45°.

If nonsurgical management is unsuccessful, surgical management includes an FDL tendon transfer procedure combined with a medial translating calcaneal osteotomy (MCO). This procedure has been determined in biomechanical and clinical studies to give good results.[14] In all surgical cases, tightness of the gastrocsoleus mechanism should be assessed and lengthening undertaken as needed.

Stage R-IIb: severe deformity

Stage R-IIb deformity displays a Meary's angle on the lateral radiograph of greater than 30° (**Fig. 1**A), talonavicular uncoverage greater than 40%, and an incongruency angle greater than 45° on the AP radiograph (see **Fig. 1**B).[10,13–15] The deformity progresses because of stretching of the secondary arch restraints such as the spring ligament, which traverses from the medial calcaneus to the navicular tuberosity.[16] Two bands make up the spring ligament: a dorsal band, which prevents abduction of the navicular, and a plantar band, which supports the talar head inferiorly. In stage R-IIb, some feet will develop more vertical collapse of the talar declination (increased apex plantar Meary's angle) than abduction deformity seen as talar head uncoverage on the AP radiograph (or vice versa) depending on whether there is more involvement of the plantar or dorsal band of the spring ligament, respectively.

If surgery is indicated, joint salvaging procedures can usually be performed. This procedure would include an FDL tendon transfer combined with a realignment procedure. Biomechanical studies have demonstrated that an MCO procedure is not adequate to correct or maintain the alignment of the rearfoot in these advanced deformities.[10,15,17] Additional procedures required to correct the deformity would include lateral column bone block lengthening procedures (calcaneal neck osteotomy or through the calcaneocuboid joint with an arthrodesis), medial column stabilizing procedures, and potentially a combination of the previously mentioned procedures with an MCO and/or a subtalar arthroereisis distraction procedure. Additionally a lateral soft tissue release, such as releasing or lengthening the peroneus brevis tendon, can be added to correct the deformity. In the most severe deformities, a

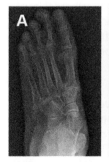
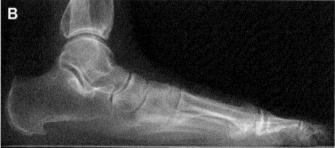

Fig. 1. Lateral (*A*) and AP (*B*) radiographs of a patient with R2b (rearfoot flexible planovalgus with greater than 50% talar head uncoverage), A1a (no ankle abnormality), and M2b (midfoot instability as seen by booking open of the first tarsometatarsal joint on the lateral view).

combination of these procedures may be needed.[18] These procedures and choices are discussed elsewhere in this issue.

In stage R-IIb patients, the spring ligament should be assessed, and if torn should be repaired or reconstructed.[17,19,20]

Stage R-III

Stage R-III deformities are rigid and not passively correctable due to arthritis or arthrosis of the rearfoot joints. Deformity is usually more chronic in nature, and patients will frequently have more pain laterally than medially over the PTT. This pain is due to impingement between the distal fibula and the valgus calcaneus, as well as subtalar joint arthritic pain. Differentiating between stages is again dependent on the degree of deformity.

Nonsurgical corrective procedures are usually not successful in arthritic deformities. Nonsurgical management is therefore limited to long-term brace immobilization with a molded ankle foot orthosis.

Stage R-IIIa: moderate fixed deformity

Stage R-IIIa, moderate fixed deformity, may be more difficult to quantify but exists when the surgeon believes that the deformity can be adequately corrected with a triple arthrodesis. An in situ arthrodesis should never be performed, and deformity correction is mandatory when preforming this procedure. In these patients, limited forefoot abduction and vertical collapse of the arch is present and can be corrected by taking down the joints, bony preparation, and realignment as part of the triple arthrodesis.

Surgical management involves a triple arthrodesis with a gastrocsoleus-Achilles lengthening as needed.

Stage R-IIIb: severe fixed deformity

With greater deformity in stage R-IIIb, additional procedures combined with a triple arthrodesis would be required to correct the deformity. Whereas angular parameters outlined in stage II can be used as a guide, individualized assessment is required, and the stage may change during treatment. The surgeon needs to be aware of the possibility of requiring these additional procedures in creating their treatment plan.

Surgical management would include a triple arthrodesis with additional deformity correction. This correction historically has been achieved with bone block resection osteotomies; however, modern correction usually combines the triple arthrodesis with either a lateral column lengthening performed through the calcaneocuboid joint or with the addition of an MCO procedure, or both. Some form of gastrocsoleus-Achilles lengthening procedure is usually required in managing these deformities.

ANKLE

Chronic and severe PTT deformity will result in progressive involvement of adjacent structures and secondary arch stabilizers. At the ankle level the deltoid ligament becomes insufficient, resulting in tibiotalar joint instability, valgus malalignment, and arthritis. This deformity was previously classified as stage IV PTT disease, but the authors believe that the ankle needs to be assessed independently of the rearfoot. Various combinations of ankle involvement with different degrees of rearfoot involvement often present, and as such treatment algorithms need to be tailored to each area separately.

Stage A-I

Stage A-I is mild deformity without loss of structural integrity of the deltoid ligament and no arthritis or bone loss at the tibial plafond.

Stage A-Ia: normal deltoid ligament

In stage A-Ia, the ankle joint remains in neutral alignment (talus and tibial plafond remain parallel). The rearfoot is managed as per its staging.

Stage A-Ib: strained deltoid ligament

In stage A-Ib, mild but passively correctable valgus (usually <5°) is seen at the ankle joint. This deformity is correctable with a reverse Coleman block-type test. The deformity will usually correct itself with an appropriate hindfoot realignment procedure, without specifically addressing the deltoid ligament itself. The rearfoot is managed as per its staging, but great care must be taken to avoid any residual valgus on completion of the procedure.

Stage A-II

Stage A-II is deltoid insufficiency with ankle valgus, without bone loss at the distal tibia.

Stage A-IIa: deltoid insufficiency without arthritic changes in the tibiotalar joint

In stage A-IIa, in addition to correcting the rearfoot deformity as per its stage, the deltoid ligament needs to be reconstructed. Various techniques for this correction are described in the literature.[2,3,13,21,22]

Stage A-IIb: deltoid insufficiency with tibiotalar arthritis

Surgical options for stage A-IIb patients include a pantalar fusion (ankle arthrodesis and triple arthrodesis) or combining a deltoid ligament reconstruction procedure with a total ankle arthroplasty. The determinate of which procedure is chosen is dependent on the degree of deformity and patient factors such as age, body mass index, and surgeon experience. The rearfoot needs to be assessed independently because in some cases a flexible deformity is present and a joint-sparing rearfoot correction can be undertaken.

Stage A-III

Stage A-III is ankle valgus associated with bone loss in the lateral tibial plafond.

Stage A-IIIa: bone loss of lateral plafond without deltoid insufficiency

With stage A-IIIa, as the talus drifts into valgus, instead of stretching out the deltoid ligament, in some cases the talus will wear away at the bone in the lateral plafond. This deformity can be seen on plane weightbearing radiographs of the ankle. As this deformity increases, more bone is lost from the plafond. Accurate assessment can be made on varus stress radiographs to determine if the deformity is correctable. If arthrodesis is used in managing these cases, care must be undertaken to correct the alignment and not to fuse the tibiotalar joint in valgus. This procedure can be accomplished by either resecting additional bone from the medial plafond (beware not to excessively shorten the limb) or by augmenting the lateral plafond with structural bone graft.

Alternatively, in these cases the ankle can be managed with an arthroplasty. In most cases the defect in the plafond is resected while preparing the distal tibia bone cuts. If a persistent defect is present, bone graft augmentation of the defect can be used. Once the trial components are placed, the deltoid competency should be assessed. In the author's (S.M. Raikin) experience, the joint is usually balanced and stable after the bony deformity is resected.

Stage A-IIIb: bone loss of the lateral plafond plus deltoid instability

In stage A-IIIb, patients can have a combination of lateral plafond bone loss and deltoid insufficiency. Deltoid integrity can be assessed on valgus stress radiographs of the ankle. If an arthrodesis is performed, the same considerations exist as is seen in stage A-IIIa. If treatment includes an ankle arthroplasty, the soft tissue ligamentous stability of the joint is assessed after trial components are inserted and the joint is balanced. This procedure can be done either by a lateral soft tissue release and using a larger polyethylene insert to balance the joint or deltoid reconstruction.

MIDFOOT

As our understanding of the AAFF has increased, so has our awareness of the involvement of the midfoot. Whereas the supination and abduction deformity most commonly occurs at the transverse tarsal joints (Chopart joints), this deformity may also develop from the midfoot. It remains unclear if collapse and supination of the midfoot occurs as a primary deformity or secondary to the chronic planovalgus deformity and attritional changes of the secondary stabilizers of the arch. These levels include the navicular-cuneiform and tarsometatarsal (TMT) articulations. Each of these levels needs to be assessed independently, both to each other and to the rearfoot and ankle. Great variation in the degree of midfoot involvement is seen clinically, without following any specific pattern relative to the rearfoot deformity.

Clinical assessment is performed by assessing the midfoot and forefoot secondary supination or varus after correcting the rearfoot alignment. This supination should be passively correctable in the normal forefoot. Additionally, weightbearing radiographs should be assessed for evidence of midfoot joint instability and arthritis.

In some situations, the deformity is able to be corrected passively only when the ankle is in a plantarflexed position. In this situation, the deformity is secondary to a tight gastrocsoleus-Achilles mechanism and is managed with a lengthening procedure.

Stage M-I

In stage M-I, a neutral or passively correctable (mild) supination or forefoot varus is present.

Stage M-Ia: neutral midfoot

In stage M-Ia, no supination of the midfoot occurs when the hindfoot is passively corrected. No additional management is required.

Stage M-Ib: mild correctable supination

In stage M-Ib, in most cases, no additional management is required. The addition of a medial forefoot post to pre- or postoperative orthotic inserts can be used to balance the deformity if needed.

Stage M-II

With stage M-II, a midfoot supination deformity occurs with correction of the rearfoot alignment (either passively in a flexible deformity or after correction of a rigid deformity with a triple arthrodesis). When ambulating, the foot will always try to create a plantigrade posture. If the midfoot supination is not corrected, the rearfoot will be forced back into a valgus alignment recreating the planovalgus deformity or overloading the lateral column resulting in pain and treatment failure.[23]

Stage M-IIa: radiographically normal articulations

The stage M-IIa deformity is due to loss of secondary arch restraints and accommodation of the midfoot to the chronic hindfoot deformity. Radiographic and clinical evaluation of the midfoot detects no abnormalities. This result is commonly seen with stage R-IIb deformities and in severe adolescent onset flexible flatfoot deformities.

Surgical correction will require a dorsal opening wedge osteotomy of the medial cuneiform, as described by Cotton,[24] to the rearfoot deformity correction. This procedure will plantarflex the medial column, thereby correcting the supination deformity and creating a balanced plantigrade foot.[25] The osteotomy is performed at the midpoint of the medial cuneiform. The plantar cortex should be left intact, while the dorsal aspect is distracted and a wedged tricortical graft or graft substitute is inserted to maintain the alignment.[26,27]

Stage M-IIb: midfoot joint instability (without arthritis)

With stage M-IIb, medial column instability can occur at the navicular-cuneiform or more frequently through the first TMT joint. This deformity can be assessed clinically but is best confirmed on assessment of the lateral weightbearing radiographs. This deformity is seen as either sagging at the affected articulation or plantar gapping (booking open) of the joint.

Surgical correction of the supination needs to be performed in addition to the rearfoot correction. In mild cases a Cotton osteotomy will correct the instability pattern, but in most cases an arthrodesis of the affected joint (navicular-cuneiform or first TMT joint) is required. It is important to adequately plantarflex the affected joint during the procedure to correct the supination and create a plantigrade foot.

Stage M-III

In stage M-III, midfoot arthritis may be secondary to midfoot instability or chronic deformity. Additionally, primary or posttraumatic arthritis of the midfoot may result in midfoot collapse and planus deformity. This condition may in turn stress the rearfoot and subsequently lead to failure of the PTT and a planovalgus (rearfoot) deformity.

Stage M-IIIa: first TMT arthritis

In stage M-IIIa, isolated arthritic involvement of the first TMT joint needs to be addressed with an arthrodesis of this articulation, regardless of the degree of instability that may or may not be present.

Stage M-IIIb: multiple joint TMT arthritis

Stage M-IIIb is usually associated with a greater degree of midfoot collapse and abduction deformity. This deformity will most commonly involve the medial and middle columns of the midfoot (first, second, and third TMT joint). The deformity may occur secondary to PTT dysfunction, but it may be primarily due to midfoot disease such as post Lisfranc injury collapse and arthritis, rheumatoid or degenerative midfoot collapse and arthritis, or neuroarthropathic collapse (**Fig. 2**). Overall clinical deformity may mimic that of a hindfoot/PTT-driven flatfoot (**Fig. 3**), but these levels need to be assessed and managed separately.

Surgical treatment involves a midfoot arthrodesis (usually including the medial three TMT joints and intercuneiform joints) with deformity correction. Correction can

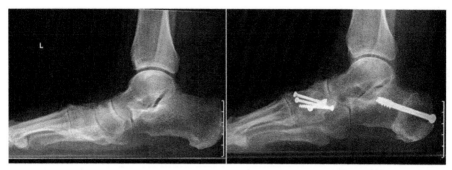

Fig. 2. Lateral radiograph demonstrating a flatfoot, with a normal hindfoot alignment (talus–first metatarsal axis). The collapse is through the unstable arthritic midfoot (R1aA1aM3b).

usually be obtained by joint mobilization and realignment prior to fusion, but an osteotomy and wedge resection may be needed to adequately correct the alignment. When a wedge resection is required, this procedure is usually a plantar and medial closing wedge resection. If rearfoot and/or ankle deformity is additionally present (either as the primary underlying pathologic condition, or secondary to the midfoot collapse) this deformity should additionally be corrected as described previously. This correction can be done at the same time or as a staged procedure. Correction of the deformity in both planes (supination and abduction) with the arthrodesis is essential to balance the foot and prevent recurrence and pain. If a combined triple arthrodesis and midfoot fusion is required, patients should be warned about the significant stiffness that will occur in the foot and risk of adjacent segment arthritic development.

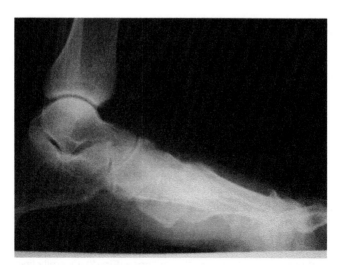

Fig. 3. Pre- and postoperative lateral radiographs of a patient with R2aA1aM3b deformity. Note the nonarthritic hindfoot sag with an apex plantar talar–first metatarsal axis, combined with the severe collapse at the navicular cuneiform articulation. Following a medializing calcaneal osteotomy, flexor tendon transfer and a navicular-cuneiform fusion, the deformity is corrected to normal.

The authors recommend that a stiff-soled rockerbottom shoe be used after correction to limit the effect of this extensive procedure.

DISCUSSION

The clinical entity of acquired flatfoot in the adult population is rather common. It may present as a new-onset unilateral flatfoot or may be due to progression of a congenital pes planovalgus. Dysfunction of the PTT is the most common cause of this condition. The various stages of tendon pathology have been clearly defined, as well as an algorithm of management.

As our understanding of the AAFF has evolved, so has the acceptance that there are other components to the deformity in addition to the PTT. The differential diagnosis of the acquired flatfoot includes traumatic dislocation of the midfoot ligaments with resultant evolution of posttraumatic arthritis, TMT osteoarthritis, inflammatory arthritis, neuropathic arthropathy, tarsal coalition, spring ligament injuries, plantar fascial rupture, proximal limb valgus, and the sequelae of neuromuscular disease. An understanding of the causes and the location(s) of pathologic conditions is critical to the successful management of this condition.

Current classification systems do not take these other causes and components of the flatfoot deformity into account or that deformity progression is not always a linear process and may affect the rearfoot, ankle, and midfoot in varying degrees and sometimes in unpredictable patterns. To that end, the RAM classification evaluates and grades each deformity by location, both clinically and radiographically (see **Table 1**). For consistency reasons, the authors have maintained the I-III grading system and the (a)/(b) subclassification scheme but have applied them to each location of potential involvement.

In creating treatment-directed algorithms, each anatomic location is assessed independently of each other, thereby allowing customized patient-specific interventions to be chosen and used. For example, a patient with a stage IIb rearfoot deformity may or may not have midfoot involvement and needs to be independently assessed for the possible addition of a midfoot procedure. Additionally, not every patient with ankle joint involvement and a flatfoot has rigid rearfoot deformity as suggested by the prior stage IV description. In certain situations a flexible rearfoot could be addressed with tendon transfers and osteotomies, while addressing the ankle via an independent decision tree with an arthroplasty or arthrodesis as needed. Finally, some patients may have a greater degree of midfoot involvement and collapse, with a strong PTT, and require only or predominantly a midfoot procedure.

In determining the recommended treatment procedure, the prior biomechanical and clinical literature has been carefully evaluated. Procedures should be tailored to address each level of the deformity, and here the authors provide a treatment algorithm. Specifics of the procedures involved are discussed elsewhere in this issue.

SUMMARY

In summary, prior classifications have provided broad guidelines for treating the AAFF without accounting for case-specific variables in determining a treatment plan. The current system breaks down the deformity into three independent levels of involvement: the rearfoot, the ankle, and the midfoot. Via a simple, easy to remember, and reproducible schema based off the original Johnson and Strom classification, each level can be independently evaluated and a patient-specific surgical treatment plan can be formulated based on our most current understanding of the AAFF.

REFERENCES

1. Beals TC, Pomeroy GC, Manoli A. Posterior tibial tendon insufficiency: diagnosis and treatment. J Am Acad Orthop Surg 1999; 7(2):112–8.
2. Bluman EM, Myerson MS. Stage IV posterior tibial tendon rupture. Foot Ankle Clin 2007;12(2):341–62.
3. Bluman EM, Title CI, Myerson MS. Posterior tibial tendon rupture: a refined classification system. Foot Ankle Clin 2007;12(2):233–49.
4. Funk DA, Cass JR, Johnson K. Acquired adult flat foot secondary to posterior tibial-tendon pathology. J Bone Joint Surg Am 1986;68(1):95–102.
5. Hill K, Saar W, Lee T, et al. Stage II flatfoot: what fails and why. Foot Ankle Clin 2003;8(1):91–104.
6. Mankey M. A classification of severity with an analysis of causative problems related to the type of treatment. Foot Ankle Clin 2003;8(3):461–71.
7. Coetzee JC, Castro MD. The indications and biomechanical rationale for various hindfoot procedures in the treatment of posterior tibialis tendon dysfunction. Foot Ankle Clin 2003;8(3):453–9.
8. Ellis SJ, Yu JC, Williams BR, et al. New radiographic parameters assessing forefoot abduction in the adult acquired flatfoot deformity. Foot Ankle Int 2009; 30(12):1168–76.
9. Haddad SL, Myerson MS, Younger A, et al. Symposium: adult acquired flatfoot deformity. Foot Ankle Int 2011;32(1):95–111.
10. Benthien RA, Parks BG, Guyton GP, et al. Lateral column calcaneal lengthening, flexor digitorum longus transfer, and opening wedge medial cuneiform osteotomy for flexible flatfoot: a biomechanical study. Foot Ankle Int 2007;28(1):70–7.
11. Parsons S, Naim S, Richards PJ, et al. Correction and prevention of deformity in type ii tibialis posterior dysfunction. Clin Orthop Relat Res 2010;468(4):1025–32.
12. Myerson MS. Adult acquired flatfoot deformity: treatment of dysfunction of the posterior tibial tendon. Instr Course Lect 1997;46:393–405.
13. Ellis SJ, Williams BR, Wagshul AD, et al. Deltoid ligament reconstruction with peroneus longus autograft in flatfoot deformity. Foot Ankle Int 2010;31(9):781–9.
14. Vora AM, Tien TR, Parks BG, et al. Correction of moderate and severe acquired flexible flatfoot with medializing calcaneal osteotomy and flexor digitorum longus transfer. J Bone Joint Surg Am 2006;88(8):1726–34.
15. Logel KJ, Parks BG, Schon LC. Calcaneocuboid distraction arthrodesis and first metatarsocuneiform arthrodesis for correction of acquired flatfoot deformity in a cadaver model. Foot Ankle Int 2007;28(4):435–40.
16. Jennings MM, Christensen JC. The effects of sectioning the spring ligament on rearfoot stability and posterior tibial tendon efficiency. J Foot Ankle Surg 2008;47(3): 219–24.
17. Williams BR, Ellis SJ, Deyer TW, et al. Reconstruction of the spring ligament using a peroneus longus autograft tendon transfer. Foot Ankle Int 2010;31(7):567–77.
18. Mosier-LaClair S, Pomeroy G, Manoli A 2nd. Operative treatment of the difficult stage 2 adult acquired flatfoot deformity [review]. Foot Ankle Clin 2001;6(1):95–119.
19. Choi K, Lee S, Otis JC, et al. Anatomical reconstruction of the spring ligament using peroneus longus tendon graft. Foot Ankle Int 2003;24(5):430–6.
20. Johnson JE, Cohen BE, DiGiovanni BF, et al. Subtalar arthrodesis with flexor digitorum longus transfer and spring ligament repair for treatment of posterior tibial tendon insufficiency. Foot Ankle Int 2000;21(9):722–9.
21. Deland JT, de Asla RJ, Segal A. Reconstruction of the chronically failed deltoid ligament: a new technique. Foot Ankle Int 2004;25(11):795–9.

22. Jeng CL, Bluman EM, Myerson MS. Minimally invasive deltoid ligament reconstruction for stage IV flatfoot deformity. Foot Ankle Int 2011;32(1):21–30.

23. Scott AT, Hendry TM, Iaquinto JM, et al. Plantar pressure analysis in cadaver feet after bony procedures commonly used in the treatment of stage II posterior tibial tendon insufficiency. Foot Ankle Int 2007;28(11):1143–53.

24. Cotton, FJ. Foot statics and surgery. N Engl J Med 1936:214:353–62.

25. Lutz M, Myerson M. Radiographic analysis of an opening wedge osteotomy of the medial cuneiform. Foot Ankle Int 2011;32(3):278–87.

26. Hirose CB, Johnson JE. Plantarflexion opening wedge medial cuneiform osteotomy for correction of fixed forefoot varus associated with flatfoot deformity. Foot Ankle Int 2004;25(8):568–74.

27. Tankson CJ. The Cotton osteotomy: indications and techniques [review]. Foot Ankle Clin 2007;12(2):309–15, vii.

The Calcaneo-Stop Procedure

F.G. Usuelli, MD*, U. Alfieri Montrasio, MD

KEYWORDS
- Flatfoot deformity • Arthroereisis • Pediatric • Adults

KEY POINTS
- The techniques used to correct flatfoot deformity can be grouped into three categories: soft tissue, bone (osteotomies and arthrodesis) and arthroereisis.
- Arthroereisis procedures were originally designed for pediatric treatment and generally involve joint-sparing techniques that correct the flatfoot deformity while preserving foot function.
- The subtalar joint could be compared with a reverse hip, called *coxa pedis*, according to Pisani.
- Calcaneo-stop is a minimally invasive procedure that acts at the center of rotation angulation of the deformity in a constraint structure.
- Calcaneo-stop is a procedure with both biomechanical and proprioceptive properties. It is designed for pediatric treatment. Theoretically it can be applied to adults if combined with other procedures to obtain a stable plantigrade foot, but medium-term follow-up studies are missing.

Flexible flatfoot is one of the most common deformities of the human body.[1] Whereas this condition is sometimes asymptomatic, it can also cause pain, difficulty walking, and physical impairment.[2]

The techniques used to correct this deformity can be grouped into three procedure categories: soft tissue, bone (osteotomies and arthrodesis) and arthroereisis.[3] The first (soft tissue) should always be combined with bone or arthroereisis, inasmuch as a stable, lasting correction is rarely obtained with the application of the soft tissue procedure alone.[4] Arthroereisis procedures were originally designed for pediatric treatment and generally involve joint-sparing techniques that correct the flatfoot deformity while preserving foot function.[5] This approach stems from extraarticular subtalar arthrodesis, first described by Grice[6] in 1952 "for correction of paralytic flatfeet in children," striving to correct the deformity without stunting foot growth.[7] A number of poor results, however, were seen with Grice's original technique because grafting a block of corticocancellous bone harvested from tibia or iliac crest was

CTS Foot and Ankle, IRCCS Galeazzi, Via R. Galeazzi 4, IT20161 Milan, Italy
* Corresponding author.
E-mail address: fusuelli@gmail.com

Foot Ankle Clin N Am 17 (2012) 183–194
doi:10.1016/j.fcl.2012.03.001
1083-7515/12/$ – see front matter © 2012 Elsevier Inc. All rights reserved.

difficult to perform.[8] The risks associated with this technique were having a graft slip out of position postoperatively resulting in the recurrence of the valgus deformity or, to fit the graft tightly, the hindfoot being forced into a varus position resulting in overcorrection.[9]

The most significant modification of the Grice technique was devised by Batchelor, with a fibular peg inserted blindly from the talus neck through the sinus tarsi,[10] but this technique resulted in a high nonunion rate.[11]

Dennyson and Fulford[12] then devised something very close to arthroereisis procedures, substituting the fibular graft with a screw and placing cancellous bone graft into the sinus tarsi, with a union rate of 95%. In any case, this technique was still an extraarticular fusion rather than a mechanical stop.[12]

Haraldsson[13] and Lelievre[14] first pointed out the possibility of blocking the sinus tarsi, restricting subtalar motion avoiding any fusions.[15] This technique is the birth of the arthroereisis procedures, with Lelievre introducing the term *lateral arthroereisis* for a temporary staple across the subtalar joint.[14]

Since then, two different approaches for this same procedure have been developed. On one side, Subotnick[16] initially described an endo sinus tarsi implant using a block of silicone elastomer, followed by Viladot's[15] popular technique of using a cup-shaped silicone implant, having a reported success rate of 99% in 234 patients. Finally, many different implants in very different shapes and materials are being designed and used. Vogt recently classified the implants as self-locking wedges, axis-altering implants, and impact-blocking devices.[17]

On the other hand, Recaredo[18] developed an eso sinus tarsi technique for limiting motion in the subtalar joint: the calcaneo-stop procedure. He inserted a cancellous screw into the calcaneus bone to interfere with talus movement in proximity of the screw head. The entry point was located in the sinus tarsi. Magnan and colleagues[19] reported 83% good results in 475 cases with 12 to 112 months follow-up time with this procedure.

Castaman[20] described a modification of this technique using a cancellous screw inserted into the talus (anterograde calcaneo-stop) with Roth[21] reporting excellent results in 48 children (94 feet) in 91.5% of the patients with a 5-year average follow-up.

An interesting phenomenon described for both endo sinus tarsi arthroereisis[22] and eso sinus tarsi calcaneo-stop[23] procedures is the maintenance of the correction even after hardware removal. It is likely that this finding had biomechanics and neuroproprioception explanations.

BIOMECHANICS

It is important to understand that flexible flatfoot is a normal foot shape, present in many infants and adults.[24] There is no consensus among health care providers as to whether flatfoot represents a deformity or a variation of normal foot shape.[25] What is clear is that the arch elevates spontaneously in most children during the first decade,[26] with no evidence of treatment efficacy for shoe modifications and insoles.[27] In fact, Helfet[28] stated that insoles could even be dangerous, leading to dependency or what he called a "life sentence" with long-term negative psychological effects, according to Driano.[29]

Although "the child foot is not just a smaller version of the adult foot" and the causes are numerous in the pediatric population,[30] the pathomechanics, over time, are comparable with adult-acquired flatfoot deformities.[2]

In this light, Scarpa's[31] observations of nearly 200 years ago are really quite interesting, noting similarities between subtalar and hip joints. He compared the acetabulum to the so-called acetabulum pedis, made up of navicular, spring ligament and anteromedial and anterolateral calcaneal subtalar articular facets. The hip is, of course, a pure ball-and-socket joint with one central rotation between two bones with an intraarticular ligament and an articular capsule, whereas the subtalar joint is not. In any case, embryologic and histologic reasons drove Pisani[32] to stress this idea, introducing the term *coxa pedis*, which describes the subtalar joint as a reverse hip.

In fact, the stable structure in the hip is the acetabulum (the socket), whereas that of the subtalar joint is the talus (the ball). Furthermore, Pisani described a medial peritalar instability with posterior tibial tendon dysfunction as being both a possible cause and consequence of spring ligament injuries, referring to them as *degenerative glenopathy*.[33] The acetabulum pedis presents a panniculus adiposus in the middle and, then, medially the bone structure with navicular posterior facet and calcaneal anterior facets. In between them it is possible to identify a glenoidlike fibrocartilage on which superomedial and plantar branches of the spring ligaments converge. In this system, the superficial branch of the deltoid ligament and the insertional portion of the posterior tibial tendon act as strengthening elements for the glenoid, laterally completed by the calcaneonavicular branch of the bifurcate (Chopart) ligament.[34] This model is consistent according to Basmajian and Stecko's[35] findings. Their electromyographic studies previously showed intrinsic static bone-ligament foot stability with no muscle activity for structural integrity, later confirmed in studies by Mann[36] and Inman.[37]

Although the foot is not a single bone, Paley's[38] concept of the center of rotation of angulation (CORA) of the deformity can be applied to the foot as well. Considering that, in flatfoot deformities, the intersection site of talus and first metatarsal axis happen mostly at talonavicular joint, biomechanically the calcaneo-stop procedure acts at the CORA of the deformity.

According to Pisani's theory, Koutsogiannis-Myerson calcaneal medial displacement osteotomy[39] is comparable to Chiari's pelvis osteotomy,[3] whereas a successful arthroereisis procedure for the hip is still missing. This result represents the success factor of this minimal invasive procedure, especially considering Nigg's[40] biomechanics study.

In fact, Benno Nigg confuted the old podiatric idea that ground reaction forces on the forefoot significantly affect foot function according to the position of the oblique Lisfranc joint axis,[41] subsequently applying the concept of rigid body rotating around subtalar joint axis to the foot complex.[42] This theory fits for every structure whose component deformations are insignificant compared with the motion of the entire structure as one entity.

A similar model closely reflects Huson's theory, which describes tarsal movement mechanism as a constraint type, later confirmed by the three-dimensional kinematics study by Cornwall and McPoil[43] and by stereophotogrammetry studies by Van Langelaan Benin and Lindberg, and Svensson.[44]

Hence, biomechanically speaking, calcaneo-stop is a minimally invasive procedure that acts at the CORA of the deformity in a constraint structure.

Neuroproprioception

Many investigators claim a proprioceptive function for the calcaneo-stop procedure,[2,4,15,19,20,23] emphasizing proof that with this active self-correction there is weak screw penetration in the calcaneus and a relatively small percentage of screw breakage, compared with what can be expected from a purely passive mechanical mechanism.

Similar observations find their scientific explanation in Japanese neurohistologic studies.[45] Neural structures were found in 22 cadaveric feet, after gold chloride impregnation. Most of these structures were free nerve endings for nociception, but it was also possible to identify mechanoreceptors as Pacini, Golgi, and Ruffini corpuscles.

An active self-correction could be also a good reason for Pisani's observation of contralateral side deformity improvement in patients treated monolaterally, especially after the recent description of a new population of cortical neurons: the mirror neurons.[46]

This special group of neuronal cells can be activated by any external stimulus (such as sight stimulus, but even proprioceptive stimulus) and facilitates adaptive active changing in the whole body. However, this is still a hypothesis. The authors advocate further studies to better acknowledge this one last principle.

SURGICAL INDICATIONS
Pediatrics

There are no controlled prospective studies showing the avoidance of long-term pain or disability by prophylactic nonoperative or operative treatment of asymptomatic flatfoot.[3]

There is, on the contrary, an abundance of studies advocating the absolute inefficiency of conservative treatments (shoe modifications and insoles) for correction of flatfoot deformity, with the exception of heel cord stretching exercise in case of concomitant Achilles brevis.[27,28,29] Furthermore, according to Morley,[3] nearly 100% of 2-year-old children are flatfooted, with a drop to 4% at age 10. This incidence makes it even more difficult to choose the correct timing in the decision-making process.

Nowadays the problem for the physician is more difficult than in the past. The choice is no longer between conservative and surgical treatment, but whether to treat the patient or not, and, if so, when.

As in the past, clinical features are more important than any other assessment. Radiographs should not dictate treatment,[3] even with abnormal values. Whereas radiographs are effective in defining static relationship between bones, absolutely no information on pain, flexibility, or function is provided.

Orthopedic surgeons share the opinion that surgical indication rate should be around 4% of the entire pediatric flexible flatfoot population, with symptomatic flexible flatfoot being candidates for surgery.[3,4] Clinical assessment should be focused on deformity reducibility, which can also be addressed by bilateral and single heel rise test and by Jack test.[2,3]

The Silfverskiold test[47] is important to determine the type of any potential Achilles contracture. It is necessary to look at forefoot position with the hindfoot reduced into neutral position to assess additional surgical intervention.[22] Of course, barefoot and shoe-clad gait must be observed, paying particular attention to atypical wear patterns on shoes.[2]

Finally, the optimal timing for this surgery is debated. Good results have been reported in the 8 to 14 age group,[4,20] but Carranza and colleagues[48] suggest performing the operation around age 12 to avoid the development of cavovarus deformity in those feet operated on at a very early age, as reported by Viladot.[15] On the other hand, Roth and colleagues[4] argued that, for patients older than 14 years, not enough correction could be reached because of the limited bone growth potential.

Therefore, considering the number of variables in this decision-making progress, it is extremely important that the referring physician for these little patients and their parents be a well-trained orthopedic surgeon skilled in foot and ankle and/or in pediatrics, rather than any other health care provider.

Adults

There is scarce literature on arthroereisis procedures in adults, with most reports being related to endo sinus tarsi arthroereisis procedures. In these cases, the main concern should not be the satisfaction rate at a short-time follow-up, but the removal rate. In an adult-structured foot it is difficult to imagine a proprioceptive active correction, and it is reasonable that the biomechanical impact be predominant. Therefore, there is clearly a high risk of correction loosening due to implant removal.

According to these principles, in a study conducted on 23 adults, Needleman[5] referred to 46% of sinus tarsi pain at an average follow-up of 44 months. He reported a 39% implant removal rate with sudden improvement of functional scores and symptoms release.

Theoretically, the calcaneo-stop procedure, being completely extraarticular, should result in less biomechanical stress symptoms and presumably work better than other endo sinus tarsi arthroereisis procedures.[2] Nevertheless, this theory, as well as its surgical indications, has yet to be documented.

In any case, arthroereisis cannot be a stand-alone procedure in adults but must be considered as a CORA[38] procedure in protection of other soft tissue CORA procedures (spring ligament repairing, for instance) and associated with other procedures that address proximal and distal pathologic conditions.

IMAGING

Radiographs should not dictate the treatment in flexible flatfoot and are not necessary for diagnosis.[2] Nonetheless, they can be useful to study uncharacteristic pain, decreased flexibility, and, of course, any surgical planning.[2,3]

In the absence of weightbearing images, the radiographic relationships between the bones will not represent the true clinical deformities, making weightbearing anteroposterior, lateral, and oblique views mandatory. In fact, a calcaneonavicular coalition is best seen on the external rotation 45° oblique view, and a talonavicular tarsal coalition can be better detected on the axial view.[2,3,20] To look for accessory navicular, an internal rotation oblique view has to be done.[49]

A number of radiographic measurements have been described for the measurement of flatfoot, but the most popular is the talar-first metatarsal angle (or Meary angle). It is subtended by the line drawn through the long axis of the talus and the navicular in relation to the first metatarsal axis in the lateral view: the flatfoot has negative or a plantar apex Meary angle.[50]

The lateral view could also be useful in determining the CORA of the deformity in a modified version, even if the foot is not a single bone, as in Paley's original concept. The site of Meary angle could approximate the CORA—most often located in the head of talus or at the talonavicular joint. In these cases any arthroereisis procedure acts at the CORA of the deformity. However, the CORA can also be located more proximal to the body of the talus, indicating a skewfoot deformity—an arthroereisis procedure contraindication.[3] Otherwise, the CORA could be located more distal within the body of one of the midtarsal bones and could be better addressed by a Miller-Hoke procedure.[51,52]

On the anteroposterior view it is important to consider the percentage of talar head uncoverage, often revealing which surgical management is more fitting following surgical indication.

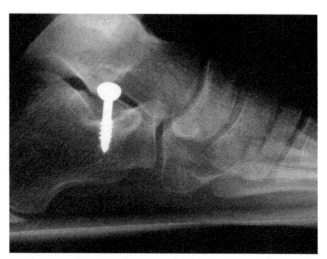

Fig. 1. Calcaneo-stop procedure.

The authors stress, in accordance with Kwon and Myerson,[2] the importance of the weightbearing views of the ankle joint to address any eventual proximal deformity and instability. Furthermore, the authors believe the hindfoot alignment should also be studied using the Saltzman and El Khoury view.[53]

Computed tomography scan and magnetic resonance imaging should be considered only for uncommon causes of flatfoot deformity such as coalition or tumor.[3]

SURGICAL TECHNIQUE
The Calcaneo-Stop Procedure

The calcaneo-stop behaves as an "internal orthotic device" and can be placed almost percutaneously with a very short recovery time and very low morbidity[2] (**Fig. 1**). Surgical treatment is usually performed under general anesthesia, with or without a tight tourniquet. A 2-cm incision is made over the sinus tarsi. Soft tissue dissection is performed bluntly, taking care to avoid the sural nerve. Under fluoroscopic control, a guide wire is vertically inserted into the calcaneus, keeping the heel well-reduced. It is 3.2-mm overdrilled. Then, a 6.5 cancellous screw is inserted. The screw should be long enough to impinge with its head against the lateral aspect of the talus preventing eversion of the subtalar joint. The common length should be around 30 to 35 mm.[4]

Anterograde Calcaneo-Stop Procedure

Castaman[20] and other investigators[4] popularized the anterograde calcaneo-stop technique with apparently a shorter incision (around 1-cm) centered on sinus tarsi (**Fig. 2**). Once the lateral process of the talus is located, under fluoroscopy, an entry hole with a trocar is performed into talus. Then a 6.5 cancellous screw is inserted at a 35°direction in the sagittal and 45° in the coronal plane. The length of the screw is similar to the original technique with the nonthreaded portion conflicting with the lateral border of the calcaneus.

Even though these two alternative techniques seem to have no significant differences regarding surgical complexity and postoperative care, the authors still recommend the traditional one based on Roth and colleagues'[4] experience describing a

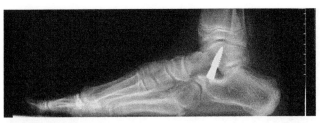

Fig. 2. Anterograde calcaneo-stop procedure.

7.45% screw malposition, posing the risk of damaging both the subtalar and ankle joints (**Figs. 3–5**).

Additional Procedures

Pediatric
In the pediatric population, the calcaneo-stop can be an isolated procedure. In fact, a passive and active correction is presumably achievable thanks to its biomechanical and proprioception properties. Furthermore, other combined procedures should address problems that frequently, but not always, are related to flatfoot. The presence of an accessory or prominent navicular should be addressed with a Kidner procedure.[54] Of course, a short Achilles tendon in children should be lengthened, preferably with a Strayer procedure.[55]

Adults
Any remodeling activity in adult hindfoot is not to be considered. Hence, the main concern should be the removal rate, which has been described by Needleman[5] for endoarthrorereisis procedures in adults at around 39%.

Theoretically, this rate should be lower in the calcaneo-stop technique. The most common complications in endorthesis, such as granuloma formation, implant displacement, biomaterial failure, tissue staining, implant irritation, and sinus tarsi pain, would not be expected with calcaneo-stop.[2] Regardless, this expectation is still a hypothesis and not a documented fact.

The authors recommend considering calcaneo-stop in adults as a possible accessory procedure to protect a medial soft tissue repairing, to be combined with any bony procedure necessary to achieve a plantigrade foot.

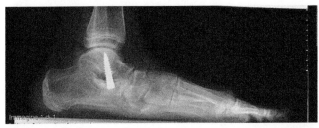

Fig. 3. Anterograde calcaneo-stop: screw malpositioning on the contralateral side of the same patient.

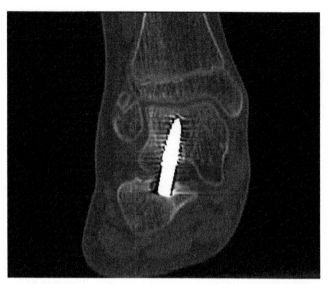

Fig. 4. Computed tomography scan: anterograde screw malpositioning (same patient).

CONTRAINDICATIONS
Pediatric

Surgical management of the flexible flatfoot is indicated for patients with pain and dysfunction. Patients not fitting this definition should not be candidates for this surgery. Therefore, the absence of pain and dysfunction is a contraindication for the calcaneo-stop procedure. In any case, not all pediatric patients will complain of the classic symptoms such as medial foot pain or lateral impingement. There is, in fact, a large spectrum of other aspecific symptoms that the physician should investigate, like shoe problems history, difficulty running, and nonspecific aches in legs.[2,3]

An inflexible flatfoot is not a surgical indication for this treatment, because it can subtend other pathologic conditions. For instance, tarsal coalition is a contraindication for the calcaneo-stop, at least as a single procedure. In these cases, a preview removal of the

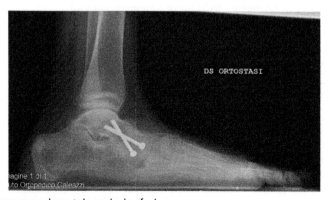

Fig. 5. Salvage procedure: talonavicular fusion.

coalition is advisable and, of course, if more than one-third of the joint is affected, a subtalar fusion would be the right choice over an arthroereisis procedure.[3]

Children outside the mentioned age group (8–14 years) represent a contraindication for this surgery. In patients undergoing the surgery too early, Viladot[15] described the risk of developing a cavovarus foot later in life. On the contrary, once the patient is too old, there is no more modeling residual potential.

Finally, both neurologic and neuromuscular diseases are contraindications.

Adults

The authors stress the idea that in adults the calcaneo-stop procedure should be combined with any other soft tissue and bone procedure to achieve a plantigrade foot, especially considering the high removal rate described for arthroereisis procedures.[4]

Considering that this procedure in some way limits subtalar joint movement, subtalar and midfoot arthritis represent a contraindication to this surgical choice for the major stress incurred after this procedure.

Rigid flatfoot and neurologic and neuromuscular diseases are absolute contraindications for this surgical treatment.

RESULTS
Pediatric

To the authors' knowledge, all published studies refer to encouraging results for the calcaneo-stop procedure in the pediatric population.[4,20] The satisfaction rate ranges between 90% and 95%, with similar results for endorthesis.[5]

All the previous studies reported a significant statistical improvement of the Meary angle around 15° with, once again, similar results for endorthesis.

Few pedographic studies are present in literature. The most relevant one available, by Kellermann and colleagues[4] shows a significant change for "relative contact time" with a postoperative increase in the lateral midfoot region (this parameter represents the actual contact time of the region divided by the contact time of the total foot in percent).

The drawback is that most of the studies have less than a 2-year follow-up—not enough to detect possible problems to the adjacent joints. Conversely, published studies on subtalar and triple arthrodesis stress transfer to adjacent joint with degenerative arthritis were not reported on prior to 10-year follow up.[3]

In addition, these implants lead to resorption of the adjacent cortical surface of the talus and calcaneus. At this time the authors cannot predict the long-term effect of this occurrence.

Some further concerns about the anterograde calcaneo-stop technique are a reported 7.45% of screw malpositioning and 2% screw penetration into the calcaneus from above with a consistent risk of subtalar damage.[4]

Adults

Short-, medium-, and long-term follow-up studies are missing.[3] To estimate the hypothetical advantage of this procedure we must to refer to endorthesis results and problems according to short-term follow-up studies. Needleman[5] refers to a lower satisfaction rate than in children (78%), with sinus tarsi pain in 46% and hardware removal in 39% at 44-month follow-up.

These studies can be explained through magnetic resonance imaging studies by Saxena and Nguyen,[56] who recently found that the tarsal canal is smaller in height and length than the implants sizes generally used. Theoretically, the calcaneo-stop technique, being totally extra sinus tarsi, should not have this problem. In any case, with such a high rate of hardware removal expected and the potential high risk of residual deformity, the calcaneo-stop procedure should be considered a procedure acting at the CORA of the deformity, to be associated with any soft tissue and bone procedures necessary to obtain a well-aligned plantigrade foot.

SUMMARY

Flexible flatfoot is one of the most common deformities. Arthroereisis procedures are designed to correct this deformity. Among them, the calcaneo-stop is a procedure with both biomechanical and proprioceptive properties. It is designed for pediatric treatment. Results similar to endorthesis procedure are reported.

Theoretically the procedure can be applied to adults if combined with other procedures to obtain a stable plantigrade foot, but medium-term follow up studies are missing.

REFERENCES

1. Pfeiffer M, Kotz R, Ledl T, et al. Prevalence of flat foot in preschool-aged children. Pediatrics 2006;118:634–9.
2. Kwon J, Myerson M. Management of the flexible flat foot in the child: a focus on the use of osteotomies for correction. Foot Ankle Clin N Am 2010;15:309–22.
3. Mosca VS. Flexible flatfoot in children and adolescents. J Child Orthop 2010;4: 107–21.
4. Roth S, Sestan B, Tudor A, et al. Minimal invasive calcaneo-stop method for idiopathic flexible per planovalgus in children. Foot Ankle Int 2007;28(9):991–5.
5. Needleman RL. Current topic review: subtalar arthroereisis for correction of flexible flatfoot. Foot Ankle Int 2005;26:336–46.
6. Grice DS. An extra-articular arthrodesis of the subastragalar joint for correction of paralytic flat feet in children. J Bone Joint Surg Am 1952;34-A:927–56.
7. Brown A. A simple method of fusion of the subtalar joint in children. J Bone Joint Surg Br 1968;50-B:369–71.
8. Pollock JH, Carrell B. Subtalar extra-articular arthrodesis in the treatment of paralytic valgus deformities: a review of 112 procedures in 100 patients. J Bone Joint Surg Am 1964;46-A:533–41.
9. Tohen A, Carmona J, Chow L, et al. Extra-articular subtalar arthrodesis: a review of 286 operations. J Bone Joint Surg Br 1969;51-B:45–52.
10. Hsu LC, Yau AC, O'Brien JP, et al. Valgus deformity of the ankle resulting from fibular resection for a graft in subtalar fusion in children. J Bone Joint Surg Am 1972;54-A: 585–94.
11. Gross RH. A clinical study of the Batchelor subtalar arthrodesis. J Bone Joint Surg Am 1976:58-A:343–9.
12. Dennyson WG, Fulford GE. Subtalar arthrodesis by cancellous grafts and metallic internal fixation. J Bone Joint Surg Br 1976;58-B:507–10.
13. Haraldsson S. Operative treatment of pes planovalgus staticus juvenilis. Acta Orthop Scand 1962;32:492–8.
14. Lelievre J. The valgus foot: current concepts and correction. Clin Orthop 1970; 70.43–55.
15. Viladot A. Surgical treatment of the child's flatfoot. Clin Orthop 1992;283:34–8.
16. Subotnick S. The subtalar joint lateral extra-articular arthroereisis: a follow-up report. J Am Podiatry Assoc 1977;32:27–33.

17. VanAman S, Schon L. Subtalar arthroereisis as adjunct treatment for the type II posterior tibial tendon insufficiency. Techniques in Foot Ankle Surgery 2006;5: 117–25.
18. Alvarez R. Calcaneo stop. Tecnica personal para el tratamiento quirurgico del pie plano-valgo del nino y adolescente joven. In: Epeldelgui T, editor. Pie plano y anomalias del antepie [in Spanish]. Madrid (Spain): Madrid Vicente; 1995. p. 174–7.
19. Magnan B, Baldrighi C, Papadia D. Flatfeet: comparison of surgical techniques. Result of study group into retrograde endorthesis with calcaneus-stop. Ital J Pediatr Orthop 1997;13:28–33.
20. Nogarin L. Retrograde endorthesis. Ital J Pediatr Othop 1997;13:34–9.
21. Kellerman P, Roth S, Gion K, et al. Calcaneo-stop procedure for paediatric flexible flatfoot. Acta Orthop Trauma Surg 2011;11:1316–3.
22. Zaret DI, Myerson MS, Arthroereisis of the subtalar joint. Foot Ankle Clin 2003;8: 605–17.
23. Pisani G. About the pathogenesis of the so-called adult acquired pes planus. Foot and Ankle Surg 2010;16:1–2.
24. Vanderwilde R, Staheli LT, Chew DE, et al. Measurements on radiographs of the foot in normal infants and children. J Bone Joint Surg Am 1988;70:407–15.
25. Steel MW 3rd, Johnson KA, DeWitz MA, et al. Radiographic measurements of the normal adult foot. Foot Ankle 1980;1:151–8.
26. Wenger DR, Mauldin D, Speck G, et al. Corrective shoes and inserts as treatment for flexible flatfoot in infants and children. J Bone Joint Surg Am 1989;71:800–10.
27. Helfet AJ. A new way of treating flat feet in children. Lancet 1956;1:262–4.
28. Rao UB, Joseph B. The influence of footwear on the prevalence of flat foot. A survey of 2300 children. J Bone Joint Surg Br 1992;74:525–7.
29. Driano AN, Staheli L, Staheli, LT. Psychosocial development and corrective shoewear use in childhood. J Pediatr Orthop 1998;18:346–9.
30. Richardson RS. Foreword. Foot and Ankle Clin 1998;3:13.
31. Scarpa A. A memoir on the congenital clubfeet of children, and of the mode of correcting that deformity. 1818. Edinburgh (Scotland): Archibald Constable; 1994. p. 8–15. [Trans.: Wishart JH. Clin Orthop Relat Res 1994;308:4–7.]
32. Pisani G. Peritalar destabilization syndrome (adult flatfoot with degenerative glenopathy). Foot Ankle Surg 2010;16:183–8.
33. Pisani G. La "coxa pedis" e i momenti torsionali astragalici. Chir Pied 1987;11:35–8 [in Italian].
34. Tryfonidis M, Jackson W, Mansour R, et al. Acquired adult flat foot due to isolate plantar calcaneo-navicular (spring) ligament insufficiency with a normal tibialis posterior tendon. Foot Ankle Surg 2006;14:89–95.
35. Basmajian JV, Stecko G. The role of muscles in arch support of the foot. An electromyographic study. J Bone Joint Surg Am 1963;45:1184–90.
36. Mann RA. Biomechanics of the foot and ankle. In: Mann RA, editor. Surgery of the foot. St Louis (MO): CV Mosby; 1986. p. 1–30.
37. Inman VT. The joints of the ankle. Baltimore (MD): Williams and Wilkins; 1976.
38. Paley D. Principles of deformity correction. Berlin: Springer-Verlag; 2002.
39. Koutsogiannis E. Treatment of mobile flat foot by displacement osteotomy of the calcaneus. J Bone Joint Surg Br 1971;53-B:96–100.
40. Nigg BM. Mechanics. In: Nigg BM, Herzog W, editors. Biomechanic of the muscoloskeletal system. 2nd edition. New York: John Wiley and Sons; 1994. p. 36.
41. Manter JT. Movements of the subtalar and transverse tarsal joints. Anat Rec 1941; 80:397.

42. Huson A. Functional anatomy of the foot. In: Jass MH, editor. Disorder of the foot and ankle. Philadelphia: WB Saunders; 1991. p.409.

43. Cornwall MW, McPoil TG. Three-dimensional movement of the foot during the stance phase of walking. J Am Podiatr Med Assoc 1999;89:56.

44. Kirby KA. Biomechanics of the normal and abnormal foot. J Am Podiatr Med Assoc 2000;90:30.

45. Akiyama K, Takakura Y, Tomita Y, et al. Neurohistology of the sinus tarsi and sinus tarsi syndrome. J Orthop Sci 1999;4:299–303.

46. Molenberghs P, Hayward L, Mattingley JB, et al. Activation patterns during action observation are modulated by context in mirror system areas. Neuroimage 2011 [epub ahead of print].

47. Silfverskiold N. Reduction of the uncrossed two joints muscles of the leg to one joint muscles in spastic conditions. Acta Chir Scand 1924;56:315.

48. Carranza A, Gimeno V, Gomez JA, et al. Giannini's prosthesis in the treatment of juvenile flatfoot. J Foot Ankle Surg 2000;6:11–7.

49. Malicky ES, Levine DS, Sangeorzan BJ. Modification of the Kidner procedure with fusion of the primary and accessory navicular bones. Foot Ankle Int 1999;20:53–4.

50. Meary R. On the measurement of the angle between the talus and the first metatarsal. Symposium: Le Pied Creux essential. Rev Chir Orthop 1967;53:389.

51. Hoke M. An operation for correction of extremely relaxed flat feet. J Bone Joint Surg 1931;13:773–83.

52. Miller GR. The operative treatment of the hypermobile flat-feet in the young child. Clin Orthop Relat Res 1977;122:95–101.

53. Saltzman CL, Khoury NJ. The hindfoot alignment view. Foot Ankle Int 1995;16(9): 572–6.

54. Kidner FC. The pre-hallux (accessory scaphoid) in its relation to the flat foot. J Bone Joint Surg 1929;11:831–7.

55. Strayer LM Jr. Recession of the gastrocnemius: an operation to relieve spastic contracture of the calf muscles. J Bone Joint Surg Am 1950;32-A:671.

56. Saxena A, Nguyen A. Preliminary radiographic findings and sizing implications on patients undergoing bioabsorbable subtalar arthroereisis. J Foot Ankle Surg 2007; 46(3):175–80.

Tarsal Coalitions in the Adult Population

Does Treatment Differ from the Adolescent?

Steven W. Thorpe, MD[a], Dane K. Wukich, MD[b],*

KEYWORDS

- Tarsal coalition • Symptomatic flatfoot • Evaluation • Treatment • Adults
- Adoloscents

KEY POINTS

- Genetic studies have shown possible autosomal dominant transmission with full penetrance, supporting the theory of failure in fetal development.
- Operative treatment should be reserved for those patients that have failed nonoperative treatment.
- Unlike adolescent coalitions, nonoperative treatment may be even more effective in the adult patient as many are asymptomatic or discovered after injury.
- Resection can be attempted for talocalcaneal coalitions that do not present with advanced arthrosis or significant hindfoot malalignment.

The diagnosis and treatment of tarsal coalition in the adolescent population have been well described, but there is a paucity of information regarding adult coalitions. The overall incidence, albeit rather unknown, has been stated to be less than 1%.[1–3] As a large proportion of adult coalitions are discovered incidentally, the overall incidence may be higher than previously reported.[2]

Pediatric calcaneonavicular coalitions usually present between the ages of 12 and 15 years (average 16 years), and talocalcaneal present a little later in age (average 18 years).[2–4] Coalitions become symptomatic in adolescents as they ossify, restricting subtalar motion.[5] Adult coalitions present at an average age of 40 and are often asymptomatic but can become symptomatic after trauma.[1,2,6]

The authors have nothing to disclose.
[a] Department of Orthopaedic Surgery, University of Pittsburgh Medical Center, Roesch Taylor Building, 2100 Jane Street, Suite 7100, Pittsburgh, PA 15203, USA; [b] Foot and Ankle Division, Department of Orthopaedic Surgery, University of Pittsburgh Medical Center, Kauffman Medical Building, 3471 Fifth Avenue, Suite 1010, Pittsburgh, PA 15213, USA
* Corresponding author.
E-mail address: wukichdk@upmc.edu

Foot Ankle Clin N Am 17 (2012) 195–204
doi:10.1016/j.fcl.2012.03.004
1083-7515/12/$ – see front matter © 2012 Published by Elsevier Inc.

foot.theclinics.com

Coalitions have been shown to occur from a failure of mesenchymal differentiation.[1,2,4,7] Genetic studies have shown possible autosomal dominant transmission with full penetrance, supporting the above theory of failure in fetal development.[1,2,8,9]

Calcaneonavicular (53%) and middle facet talocalcaneal (37%) coalitions are the most common, and are bilateral in 50% to 80% of patients.[2,3,8] Talonavicular and calcaneocuboid coalitions also occur but are much less common.[2] In the pediatric and adolescent population, these coalitions most commonly present as a painful, rigid flatfoot, and sometimes with associated peroneal spasm.[1] Harris and Beath[10,11] were the first to describe talocalcaneal coalitions as a cause of the peroneal spastic flatfoot. In contrast, coalitions that are diagnosed in adulthood often do not present with flatfoot or peroneal spasm.[1] The peroneal spastic flatfoot is suggestive of a coalition but is not definitive.[2,12] In an incidence study of 43 patients, Stormont and Peterson[3] reported only 2 of 60 had peroneal spasm (age range 1 week–54 years). Gonzalez and Kumar[12] demonstrated a higher association with 20 of 48 patients with calcaneonavicular coalitions manifesting peroneal spasm and a rigid flatfoot.

Adult coalitions are often asymptomatic and incidentally discovered during a workup for another unrelated foot or ankle problem. Occasionally, patients will present with sinus tarsi pain, peroneal spasm, or painful pes planus. In a retrospective series of adult coalitions by Varner and Michelson,[1] 18 (67%) of 27 coalitions were symptomatic and discovered during workup for ankle sprains, instability, and sinus tarsi pain, while the remaining 9 (33%) of 27 of coalitions were asymptomatic. In a series of active young adult patients, coalitions were discovered after strenuous activity, but most had a history of prior symptoms that were not reported.[13]

EVALUATION

The initial clinical exam should focus on any hindfoot varus or valgus deformity and whether any associated deformity is fixed or flexible. In the study by Varner and Michelson,[1] only 7 (22%) of 32 feet were found to have a pes planovalgus foot/hindfoot. Additionally, subtalar active and passive motion should be assessed and compared between both sides, as 83% of adult coalitions have decreased or absent subtalar motion on exam.[1,2] Peroneal tendons should also be evaluated for tenderness and signs of inflammation. Calcaneonavicular coalitions often present with sinus tarsi pain while talocalcaneal coalitions typically present with deep subtalar joint pain, and symptoms are often discovered after minor trauma.[2,5]

Radiographic evaluation should begin with standard weight-bearing orthogonal foot and ankle views. Weight-bearing hindfoot alignment views should also be obtained for coronal alignment. A 45° medial oblique view best demonstrates a calcaneonavicular coalition (**Fig. 1**), and a Harris axial heel view is the radiograph of choice for a suspected talocalcaneal coalition.[2,5] In the Harris axial view, the posterior and middle facets should be parallel, but greater than 25° angulation of the medial facet away from the posterior facet signifies a talocalcaneal coalition.[5] Varner and Michelson[1] reported that 94% of adult coalitions could be found on plain radiographs alone. Other radiographic features that have been shown to indicate the presence of a coalition include talar beaking in talocalcaneal coalitions, and the "anteater nose," seen on the lateral roentgenogram as an elongation of the anterior process of the calcaneus toward the navicular for a calcaneonavicular coalition, in calcaneonavicular coalitions (see **Fig. 1**).[1,2,12,14] For a talocalcaneal coalition a narrow subtalar joint space or the presence of a "C" sign on a lateral non–weight-bearing radiograph has been suggested (**Fig. 2**); however, it has been shown to lack both sensitivity and specificity.[1] The "C" sign results from the distortion of the normal talar and calcaneal

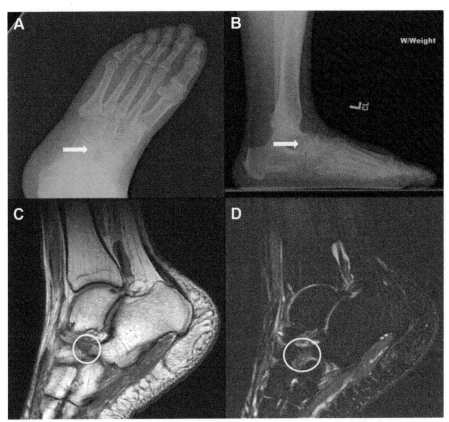

Fig. 1. (*A–D*) A 52-year-old man with left foot pain for 6 months after a fall from 20 feet. He had severe pain limiting daily and recreational activities, including difficulty with uneven ground. His pain was localized to the sinus tarsi and anterior process of calcaneus. Severe pain was elicited with passive subtalar inversion and eversion. His AOFAS was 33. (*A*) Oblique radiograph left foot demonstrating decreased space (*arrow*) between anterior process of the calcaneus and navicular. (*B*) Weight-bearing lateral radiograph of left foot demonstrating "anteater sign" (*arrow*). (*C*) T1 MRI sagittal left foot demonstrating calcaneonavicular coalition (*circle*). (*D*) T2 MRI sagittal left foot demonstrating fibrous calcaneonavicular coalition (*circle*).

alignment. This radiographic sign is created by an abnormal bony bridge between the talar dome and sustentaculum tali, medial outline of the talar dome, and the inferior outline of sustentaculum tali.[15]

Even though many coalitions can be diagnosed on standard radiographs, more advanced imaging can be useful for diagnosis and treatment. Computed tomography (CT) evaluation can better characterize bony coalitions, identifying the location and size.[2] Magnetic resonance imaging (MRI) is useful for characterizing the type of coalition, such as fibrous, cartilaginous, or osseous coalitions (see **Fig. 1**).[2] MRI is also useful when a traumatic mechanism is also involved in the onset of symptoms as it can evaluate other potential sources of pain such as osteochondral lesions, ligament disruptions, or tendon pathology. MRI is also useful as it provides visualization of bone marrow. Specifically, marrow hyperintensities in the subchondral bone

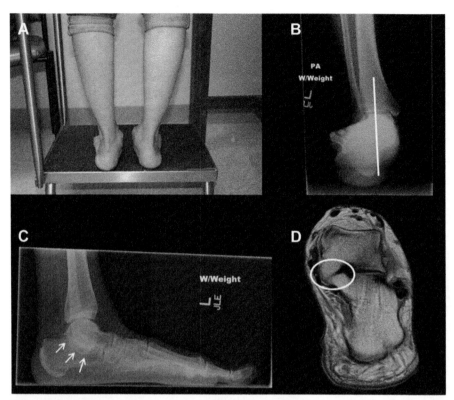

Fig. 2. (A–D) A 45-year-old woman with bilateral foot pain (left > right) for longer than 2 years. Pain primarily in the sinus tarsi region. The patient had increasing pain despite conservative treatment for 2 years with CAM walker boot and physical therapy. Her AOFAS score was 55. (A) Hindfoot view demonstrating bilateral pes planovalgus deformity. (B) Weight-bearing left hindfoot alignment view radiograph with plumb line demonstrating hindfoot valgus. (C) Weight-bearing left lateral radiograph demonstrating "C"-sign (arrows). (D) Axial T1 MRI demonstrating middle facet talocalcaneal coalition (circle).

surrounding the area of possible coalition were found to be indicative of a talocalcaneal coalition.[16]

NONOPERATIVE TREATMENT

In the adult population, a coalition usually becomes symptomatic secondary to injury at the synchondrosis or syndesmosis between the 2 bones. This is rare in the ossified coalition and is akin to a stress fracture at the bar between the 2 bones due to the limited mobility present at this area. The goal of treatment is relief of pain and decreasing tarsal stress.[1] As with pediatric tarsal coalitions, the treatment of adult tarsal coalitions begins with nonoperative treatment. This includes activity modification, physical therapy, University of California Biomechanics Laboratory orthoses, nonsteroidal anti-inflammatory drugs (nsaids), and short leg cast immobilization for 4 to 6 weeks.[1,2] Most coalitions are asymptomatic prior to recent trauma, and thus, a nonoperative treatment protocol may be effective.[2,8] Cowell[17] demonstrated 25% to 30% success with a short-leg walking cast for a 6-week period in pediatric patients.

The few studies on adult coalitions have reported an 18% to 67% efficacy from nonoperative treatment only.[1,18] In the study by Varner and Michelson,[1] of those patients with a symptomatic coalition, 6 (33%) of 18 patients failed nonoperative treatment; however, it is difficult to determine a true efficacy of nonoperative management in adults due to a lack of evidence and an unknown prevalence of asymptomatic cases. Other questions that remain unanswered include defining the natural history of asymptomatic tarsal coalitions and whether there any indications for operative treatment for the asymptomatic coalitions.

OPERATIVE TREATMENT

Operative treatment should be reserved for those patients who have failed nonoperative treatment, although the duration of such treatment is not well defined. The goals of operative treatment are pain relief and restoration of more normal subtalar kinematics.[19] In the ideal setting, restoration of subtalar kinematics is an important goal of resections; however, significant improvement in kinematics may not occur after coalition resection despite significant improvements in American Orthopaedic Foot and Ankle Society (AOFAS) hindfoot scores and passive subtalar inversion and eversion.[19] The decision for surgical treatment can be complex because of the wide variety in presentation.[20] Most pediatric coalitions are treated with resection of the coalition and interposition with either fat graft, extensor digitorum brevis (EDB), as in the case of calcaneonavicular coalition[21] or flexor hallucis longus for talocalcaneal coalitions.[21,22]

Favorable results have been shown for calcaneonavicular coalition excision in the adolescent.[2,23] The need for interposition grafting after coalition excision is difficult to determine, and results can be conflicting as to what type of graft is best.[2,20,21,23,24] A recent retrospective review by Mubarak and colleagues[24] found excellent outcomes in 87% of patients treated with excision and fat interposition grafting. Regrowth of the coalition was found in only 13%, and they reported a preference for fat interposition, rather than EDB, as the EDB was not large enough to fill the defect and resulted in a less satisfactory wound appearance.[24] Talonavicular beaking, originally thought to be an indicator of arthrosis and poor results, has not been shown to be a contraindication to excision.[2,12,18,20,25] More classic signs of arthritis have been described as criteria in favor of triple arthrodesis instead of excision.[2,18,20,26] Long-term follow-up studies have shown good or excellent results into adulthood for 69% of patients who undergo excision of calcaneonavicular bars.[25]

The surgical treatment of talocalcaneal coalition is much more controversial in regards to excision versus arthrodesis.[26] Hindfoot valgus, specifically valgus greater than 21°, has been shown to be predictive of a poor outcome after excision, but talar beaking has not been shown to affect outcomes.[2,27,28] Again, graft interposition has a variety of evidence that is inconclusive as to type, source, and even the need for it.[2,6,11,22,29,30] The size of the talocalcaneal coalition has also been implicated in the decision paradigm for surgical treatment. Coalition size greater than 50% of the size of the posterior facet was shown to predict negative results after resection.[2,27,28] For this reason, Luhman and Schoenecker[27] advocated preoperative CT scans in order to determine resection versus arthrodesis. Any signs of subtalar arthrosis should be more indicative of the need for an arthrodesis procedure, whether subtalar or triple arthrodesis.[2]

OUTCOMES

The available orthopedic literature on the outcomes of the treatment of tarsal coalitions in the adult population is sparse. This body of evidence is Level IV, based

Table 1
Clinical studies of calcaneonavicular coalition (age >16 years)

First Author	Year	Level of Evidence	Number of Feet	Results/Outcomes
Varner[1]	2000	IV	14	11 feet asymptomatic (both CN and TC), 1 resection with pain-free outcome
Cohen[18]	1996	IV	13 (12 patients)	Resection and interposition successful 10/12 Unsuccessful in 2 patients: 1: hindfoot arthrodesis, 2: triple arthrodesis Complications: 5/13 (38%) feet Improvement (10°) in motion
Scott[31]	2007	IV	8 (7 patients)	Resection and EDB interposition Average postoperative AOFAS 87 (79–97) All patients would elect for surgery again 5 patients complained of only mild pain at follow-up 2/7 (29%) complications

Abbreviations: CN, calcaneonavicular; TC, talocalcaneal.

on retrospective, case series studies[1,17,31] (**Tables 1** and **2**). The studies are underpowered and lack control groups, and one of the studies does not even differentiate treatment and outcomes between calcaneonavicular and talocalcaneal coalitions.[1] Varner and Michelson[1] had only 4 patients (5 feet) treated operatively (1 resection and 4 subtalar arthrodeses) of 18 symptomatic patients. The author reported pain relief for all operative cases but failed to delineate for which coalitions a subtalar arthrodesis was performed.[1] Only one of these studies used a validated outcome measure (AOFAS hindfoot score) for postoperative assessment although preoperative scores were not reported.[31] Based on these studies, it is difficult to delineate a treatment paradigm for the adult coalition.

Table 2
Clinical studies of talocalcaneal coalition (age ≥15 years)

First Author	Year	Level of Evidence	Number of Feet	Results/Outcomes
Varner[1]	2000	IV	18	Subtalar arthrodesis (4) scheduled for subtalar arthrodesis (2) does not specify CN or TC
Scranton[6]	1987	IV	12 (8 patients)	Cast (5) – all satisfied Resections (7) Good results 6/7
Philbin[32]	2008	IV	7 (7 patients)	Resection (7) Failed resection requiring arthrodesis (1) Average change in preoperative and postoperative AOFAS scores approached significance ($P = .051$) Higher cartilaginous content of coalition associated with better outcome ($P = .016$)

Abbreviations: CN, calcaneonavicular; TC, talocalcaneal.

The treatment of adult calcaneonavicular coalition has been similar to the adolescent. The available literature shows results similar to the adolescent literature (**Table 1**). Scott and Tuten,[31] in a study of 7 adult patients (8 feet), demonstrated a postoperative average AOFAS of 87 with resection of a calcaneonavicular coalition and EDB interposition. Unfortunately, preoperative AOFAS scores were not reported. Two of the 7 patients sustained mild complications, including 1 superficial infection and 1 sural nerve dysesthesia that resolved.[31] Similar good results were reported in 12 adult patients (13 feet) who underwent resection and EDB interposition, noting successful outcomes in 10 of 12 patients with an average improvement in subtalar motion of 10°. Two patients remained symptomatic and underwent arthrodesis. Nine (75%) of the 12 patients had evidence of preoperative degenerative arthritis, and talar beaking was seen in 7 (54%) of 13 feet. The authors agreed with previous adolescent studies by Swiontkowski and colleagues[20] and Gonzales and Kumar[12] that talar beaking did not correlate with talonavicular arthrosis, and thus should not be a contraindication to coalition resection.[2,12,18,20] Despite reporting success in 10 of 12 patients, the complication rate was relatively high: 38% (5 of 13 feet). The authors attribute some of these complications to an earlier technique of EDB interposition with pull-out suture. Subsequently, patients received bone wax and Gelfoam without interposition.[18]

There is even less evidence for the treatment of talocalcaneal coalitions in adults (**Table 2**).[1,6,32] From one of these studies, it is impossible to fully delineate how talocalcaneal coalitions were treated.[1] Varner and Michelson[1] reported subtalar arthrodesis in 4 patients with an additional 2 patients scheduled for subtalar arthrodesis; however, the authors did not specify for which type of coalition these fusions were performed. Scranton[6] reviewed outcomes of operative treatment for talocalcaneal coalitions. This study involved symptomatic patients with an average age of 24 (range 11–55), and adults represented 8 of 14 patients (12 of 23 coalitions) (see **Table 2**). Only 2 of 8 adults presented with a spastic flatfoot (ages 17 and 24). The authors' treatment protocol for subtalar coalitions was dependent on the amount of joint surface involved in the coalition. If greater than 50% was involved, then a short leg cast was used for a minimum of 16 weeks. A triple arthrodesis was performed for those patients who failed nonoperative management. For those coalitions with less than 50% joint involvement, resection was performed along with interposition of fat graft from posterior to the calcaneus. Postoperative management consisted of 3 weeks in a non–weight-bearing cast, followed by an additional 3 weeks in a weight-bearing cast. Five coalitions (3 adults) which were treated in a cast achieved "satisfactory" results. Of note, 2 of these patients were asymptomatic until they presented after ankle sprain. Results were "good" for 6 of 7 coalitions (4 of 5 adults) after resection.[6] Despite apparent good results after resection, Hetsroni and colleagues[19] demonstrated that subtalar kinematics are not restored following coalition resection, which may precipitate further degenerative changes. Scranton[6] recommended that arthrodesis be performed when a coalition is "unresectable" and fails conservative treatment or if advanced arthrosis is present.

Philbin and colleagues,[32] in a more recent retrospective series of 7 patients, included the type of coalition, percent coalition, hindfoot alignment, preoperative arthritis, and age at resection in the analysis of outcomes after resection of middle facet tarsal coalition in adults. The age range included was 15 to 56 years. The authors did not include details of methods of resection and interposition, if any. They did address hindfoot valgus with a medial displacement calcaneus osteotomy in 4 of 7 cases. Gastrocnemius recession was performed in an unknown number of cases. Follow-up was fairly limited with an average of 17 months (range

7–36 months). The only variable to have a significant effect on outcome was the relative percentage of cartilaginous content in a coalition ($P = .016$) with improved outcomes with increasing cartilaginous content. One patient failed resection and required arthrodesis. Postoperative mean AOFAS scores were improved for the remaining 6 patients, but this was not significant ($P = .051$). Unfortunately, due to small sample size, the effects of hindfoot alignment, percent coalition, age, and degree of arthrosis on outcomes after resection could not be determined and were not significant.[32]

SUMMARY

There is a paucity of information on adult coalitions without large, well-designed outcome studies. Current recommendations are thus similar to those for adolescents. Based on the available literature, current recommendations include an initial trial of adequate nonoperative treatment in symptomatic coalitions. Unlike adolescent co-alitions, nonoperative treatment may be even more effective in the adult patient as many are asymptomatic or discovered after injury. If nonoperative treatment fails, then surgical intervention is considered and tailored to the location of the coalition, existing advanced arthrosis, and any existing deformity. Similar to the adolescent, surgical treatment for adult calcaneonavicular coalitions typically involves an attempt at resection with some type of interposition.

Resection can be attempted for talocalcaneal coalitions that do not present with advanced arthrosis or significant hindfoot malalignment. For those patients with advanced arthrosis, more than 50% involvement of the joint hindfoot malalignment, subtalar or triple arthrodesis is recommended. The decision between resection and arthrodesis is controversial in the adolescent population. With few outcome studies in adults, it is even more difficult to make definitive treatment recommendations; however, the indications for resection are likely even more limited. It is likely that the adult subtalar coalition that becomes symptomatic and fails nonoperative treatment will require arthrodesis for full pain relief and improvement in objective outcome measures, such as the AOFAS hindfoot score.

Our treatment algorithm focuses first on a trial of nonoperative treatment of at least 3 months regardless of coalition location. After failed nonoperative treat-ment, calcaneonavicular coalitions are in most cases treated with excision and interpositional fat graft. For talocalcaneal coalitions, resection is offered to patients with neutral hindfoot alignment, some preservation of subtalar joint motion and no adjacent joint arthrosis. The patients are advised that the outcome after resection of talocalcaneal coalitions is less predictable than resection of calcaneonavicular coalitions. Those patients with absent subtalar motion and relatively normal hindfoot alignment are candidates for in situ fusion of the subtalar joint. For those patients with greater than 15° of valgus hindfoot malalignment on a weight-bearing hindfoot alignment view or adjacent joint arthrosis, a triple arthrodesis is recommended with or without medial displacement osteotomy of the calcaneus. Adjacent joint arthrosis may be determined by radiographs, CT scan, or preoperative MRI.

REFERENCES

1. Varner KE, Michelson JD. Tarsal coalition in adults. Foot Ankle Int 2000;21:669–72.
2. Lemley F, Berlet G, Hill K, et al. Current concepts review: tarsal coalition. Foot Ankle Int 2006;27:1163–9.
3. Stormont DM, Peterson HA. The relative incidence of tarsal coalition. Clin Orthop 1983;181:28–36.

4. Jack EA. Bone anomalies of the tarsus in relation to "peroneal spastic flat foot." J Bone Joint Surg Br 1954;36:530–42.
5. Cowell HR, Elener V. Rigid painful flatfoot secondary to tarsal coalition. Clin Orthop 1983;177:54–60.
6. Scranton PE. Treatment of symptomatic talocalcaneal coalition. J Bone Joint Surg 1987;69:533–9.
7. Harris B. Anomalous structure in the developing human foot. Abstract Anat Rec 1955;121:399.
8. Leonard MA. The inheritance of tarsal coalition and its relationship to spastic flat foot. J Bone Joint Surg Br 1974;56:520–6.
9. Wray JB, Herndon CN. Hereditary transmission of congenital coalition of the calcaneus to the navicular. J Bone Joint Surg 1963;45:365–72.
10. Harris RI, Beath T. Etiology of peroneal spastic flat foot. J Bone Joint Surg Br 1948;30:624–34.
11. Salomao O, Napli MM, de Carvalho AE, et al. Talocalcaneal coalition: diagnosis and surgical management. Foot Ankle Int 1992;13:251–6.
12. Gonzales P, Kumar SJ. Calcaneonavicular coalition treated by resection and interposition of the extensor digitorum brevis muscle. J Bone Joint Surg 1990;72:71–7.
13. Rankin EA, Baker GI. Rigid flatfoot in the young adult. Clin Orthop 1974;104:244–8.
14. Oestreich AE, Mize WA, Crawford AH, et al. The "Anteater nose": a direct sign of calcaneonavicular coalition on the lateral radiograph. J Pediatr Orthop 1987;7:709–11.
15. Brown RR, Rosenberg ZS, Thornhill BA. The C sign: more specific for flatfoot deformity than subtalar coalition. Skeletal Radiol 2001;30:84–7.
16. Sijbrandij ES, van Gils APG, de Lange EE, et al. Bone marrow ill-defined hyperintensities with tarsal coalition: MR imaging findings. Eur J Radiol 2002;43:61–5.
17. Cowell HR. Talocalcaneal coalition and new causes of peroneal spastic flatfoot. Clin Orthop 1972;85:16–22.
18. Cohen BE, Davis WH, Anderson RB. Success of calcaneonavicular coalition resection in the adult population. Foot Ankle Int 1996;15:569–72.
19. Hetsroni I, Nysaka M, Mann G, et al. Subtalar kinematics following resection of tarsal coalition. Foot Ankle Int 2008;29:1088–94.
20. Swiontkowski MF, Scranton PE, Hansen S. Tarsal coalition: Long-term results of surgical treatment. J Ped Orthop 1983;3:287–92.
21. Moyes ST, Crawfurd EJP, Aichroth PM. The interposition of extensor digitorum brevis in the resection of calcanonavicular bars. J Pediatr Orthop 1994;14:387–8.
22. Raikin S, Cooperman DR, Thompson GH. Interposition of the split flexor hallucis longus tendon after resection of a coalition of the middle facet of the talocalcaneal joint. J Bone Joint Surg 1999;81:11–9.
23. Mitchell GP, Gibson JM. Excision of calcaneonavicular bar for painful spasmodic foot. J Bone Joint Surg Br 1967;49:281–7.
24. Mubarak SJ, Patel PN, Upasani VV, et al. Calcaneonavicular coalition: treatment by excision and fat graft. J Pediatr Orthop 2009;29:418–26.
25. Inglis G, Buxton RA, Macnicol MF. Symptomatic calcaneonavicular bars, the results 20 years after surgical excision. J Bone Joint Surg Br 1986;68:128–31.
26. Mosier KM, Asher M. Tarsal coalitions and peroneal spastic flat foot. J Bone Joint Surg 1984;66:976–84.
27. Luhmann SJ, Schoenecker PL. Symptomatic talocalcaneal coalition resection: indications and results. J Ped Orthop 1998;18:748–54.
28. Widhe PH, Torode IP, Dickens DR, et al. Resection for symptomatic talocalcaneal coalition. J Bone Joint Surg Br 1994;76:797–801.

29. Kumar MD, Guille JT, Lee MS, et al. Osseous and nonosseous coalition of the middle facet of the talocalcaneal joint. J Bone Joint Surg 1992;74:529–35.
30. Olney BW, Asher MA. Excision of symptomatic coalition of the middle facet of the talocalcaneal joint. J Bone Joint Surg 1987;69:539–44.
31. Scott AT, Tuten HR. Calcaneonavicular coalition resection with extensor digitorum brevis interposition in adults. Foot Ankle Int 2007;28:890–5.
32. Philbin TM, Homan B, Hill K, et al. Results of resection for middle facet tarsal coalitions in adults. Foot Ankle Spec 2008;1:344–9.

Tendon Transfer Options in Managing the Adult Flexible Flatfoot

Michael S. Aronow, MD

KEYWORDS

- Posterior tibial tendon dysfunction • Flatfoot • Tendon transfer • Posterior tibial tendon
- Tibialis posterior • Flexor digitorum longus • Flexor hallucis longus
- Peroneus brevis

KEY POINTS

- Posterior tibialis function may be compromised or associated with pain in adult patients with symptomatic flexible flatfoot deformity.
- Surgical treatment may include debridement and augmentation or replacement of the diseased posterior tibial tendon using a tendon transfer to decrease pain and attempt to restore functional hindfoot inversion strength.
- The most common tendon transferred in this situation is the flexor digitorum longus because of its anatomic proximity, in phase firing during the gait cycle, and limited functional loss if sacrificed.
- Other tendon transfers that have been described in place of the flexor digitorum longus are the flexor hallucis longus and peroneus brevis.

Posterior tibial tendon (PTT) dysfunction is a disorder in which there is a symptomatic pathologic condition involving the PTT and/or spring ligament complex. Some patients with PTT dysfunction previously had a normal or slightly cavus arch before acquiring a flexible flatfoot during adulthood. Other patients with PTT dysfunction may still have a normal or slightly cavus arch. However, more commonly there is a preexisting flatfoot that may have developed increased deformity that may be flexible or fixed. Per the Johnson and Strom classification[1] as modified by Myerson,[2] stage 1 PTT dysfunction has an intact arch, stage 2 has a flexible flatfoot deformity, stage 3 has a fixed flatfoot deformity, and stage 4 has an underlying stage 2 or stage 3

Commercial relationships: The author is a nonpaid consultant for Arthrex, Inc, which makes an interference screw shown in this article.
Department of Orthopaedic Surgery, University of Connecticut School of Medicine, Medical Arts and Research Building, 263 Farmington Avenue, Farmington, CT 06034–4037, USA
E-mail address: aronow@nso.uchc.edu

Foot Ankle Clin N Am 17 (2012) 205–226
doi:10.1016/j.fcl.2012.02.001
1083-7515/12/$ – see front matter © 2012 Elsevier Inc. All rights reserved.

deformity with the addition of valgus tilt at the ankle joint secondary to deltoid ligament laxity or lateral ankle arthritis. In many patients with stage 2 PTT dysfunction the deformity may only be correctable with the ankle in equinus or the gastrocnemius relaxed by knee flexion.

The initial treatment of patients with PTT dysfunction is usually nonoperative and includes supportive orthoses, physical therapy, antiinflammatory medications, and potentially selective injections. Should that treatment be unsuccessful, surgery may be performed to address any pathologic condition in the PTT, which is the focus of this article. Additional soft tissue procedures are often also performed. Patients with spring and/or deltoid ligament pathology may benefit from direct repair, imbrication, or graft reconstruction.[3–5] Significant triceps surae contractures should be addressed with gastrocnemius recession with a modified Baker partial soleus aponeurosis lengthening added or a tendo-Achilles lengthening substituted if there is significant equinus with the knee flexed.[6] How much triceps surae contracture is considered to be "significant" is somewhat controversial and beyond the scope of this article. Relatively hindfoot motion-sparing procedures including osteotomies, limited fusions, and subtalar arthroereisis[7] may be added to improve the arch and decrease biomechanical strain on the PTT repair, tendon transfer, and spring and deltoid ligaments. A comprehensive discussion of these procedures is also beyond the scope of this article, but they include medial displacement calcaneal osteotomy,[8,9] intracalcaneal lengthening osteotomies such as the Evans procedure,[10] Cotton medial cuneiform dorsal opening wedge osteotomy,[11] combined calcaneal osteotomies,[12] calcaneocuboid distraction arthrodesis,[13] and medial column naviculocuneiform and/or first tarsometatarsal fusions.[14] In low demand patients or patients with significant subtalar arthritis tibialis posterior it may be appropriate to add a subtalar fusion.[15]

BIOMECHANICS

The tibialis posterior is the principal supinator of the subtalar joint, an adductor of the midfoot, and an ankle plantarflexor. Through its multiple attachments on the plantar aspect of the foot the PTT also helps support the ligaments that maintain the arch of the foot. During the stance phase of normal gait the tibialis posterior fires eccentrically after heel strike allowing the hindfoot to pronate in a controlled fashion, which in turn unlocks the talonavicular and calcaneocuboid joints allowing the foot to better absorb shock. During midstance and toe-off the tibialis posterior fires concentrically to bring the foot back into supination, locking the talonavicular and calcaneocuboid joints to provide a rigid arch so that the gastrocnemius and soleus can effectively push off the forefoot. Because the PTT has a limited excursion of only 1 to 2 cm, any insult, no matter how minor, that lengthens this tendon may have an adverse effect on its function.[16] In addition to decreased hindfoot eversion strength, the diminished ability of the lengthened tibialis posterior to lock the hindfoot and stabilize the arch may lead to decreased push-off strength and difficulty with gait. However, when a pathologic condition weakens the PTT with its antagonist the peroneus brevis intact, the arch usually does not immediately become flat unless there is a concurrent significant spring ligament tear. This delay is because it takes time for the cumulative increased forces on the spring ligament and the other plantar ligaments of the foot secondary to the loss of protective effect of the eccentric firing of the tibialis posterior after heel strike to stretch out these ligaments. Therefore, theoretically it may be beneficial with respect to arch preservation to maintain or restore tibialis posterior function and provide sufficient external orthotic support to the ligaments of the foot early on in the disease process.

With respect to the biomechanical principals of tendon transfer, an excellent review was recently published by Bluman and Dowd.[17] An ideal tendon transfer would provide sufficient strength to meet the patient's needs and goals without excessive sacrifice and be performed technically in a way to maximize the transferred tendons' function and minimize morbidity. Based on the concept that relative muscle strength is proportional to cross-sectional area, Silver and colleagues[18] calculated the relative strength of the tibialis posterior to be 6.4, the tibialis anterior 5.6, the peroneus longus 5.5, the flexor hallucis longus (FHL) 3.6, the peroneus brevis 2.6, and the flexor digitorum longus (FDL) 1.8. Therefore, even without taking into account the expected associated loss of a grade of strength for a transferred tendon, the muscles typically used to reconstruct the tibialis posterior are much weaker than the one that eventually failed against at least the same biomechanical stress an isolated tendon transfer would face. Whereas the FDL and FHL are closer in strength to the principal antagonist of the PTT, the peroneus brevis, the stronger peroneus longus also acts as an evertor of the subtalar joint, and its activity begins earlier and ends later during stance phase than the peroneus brevis. Therefore, the long-term functional results of tendon transfers to the PTT might be theoretically better if adjunctive procedures were performed to decrease the biomechanical stress on the tendon transfer by improving the longitudinal arch of the foot, decreasing antagonistic hindfoot eversion force, and/or increasing total hindfoot inversion force by increasing the transferred tendon's moment arm and/or preserving the tibialis posterior muscle function when possible.

Kitaoka and colleagues[19] created a cadaver flatfoot deformity model and applied load to the plantar aspect of the foot and the Achilles, peroneus longus, peroneus brevis, posterior tibial, and FDL tendons to simulate the midstance phase of gait. They found that subtalar fusion provided significantly greater deformity correction of foot position including arch height than a Johnson and Strom[1] side-to-side FDL tendon transfer to the PTT. In a similar study,[20] the same investigators found that foot position including arch height improved substantially after deltoid ligament reconstruction but not after FDL tendon transfer. In a multisegment biomechanical flatfoot model Arangio and Salathe[21] noted that a simulated 10-mm medial displacement calcaneal osteotomy substantially decreased the load on the first metatarsal and the moment at the talonavicular joint and increased the load on the fifth metatarsal and the calcaneocuboid joint. The subsequent addition of an FDL transfer had only a small additional effect.

CLINICAL DECISION-MAKING

When operating on patients with PTT dysfunction, the surgeon needs to make two important decisions with respect to preserving PTT function. First a decision needs to be made as to whether or not the diseased PTT should be preserved or completely excised. The second decision is whether or not a tendon transfer is indicated to augment or replace the pathologic PTT and if so, which tendon and technique is used.

If the PTT has minimal tendinopathy it generally should be preserved. On the other hand, most surgeons would excise a nonfunctional PTT with severe tendinosis and scarring. There are also chronic complete ruptures in which the proximal stump of the PTT has retracted well into the leg and cannot be re-approximated to the distal tendon stump. However, controversy exists with respect to whether or not to excise or retain the PTT when there is functional tendon with associated areas of tendinosis or large chronic but repairable tear or tears. One school of thought is that the diseased PTT is a pain generator that will likely cause persistent discomfort if maintained. The other school of thought believes that the tibialis posterior is stronger than the muscle tendon units used to replace it and therefore it is in the patient's best interest not to unnecessarily sacrifice it when just addressing the areas of symptomatic tendinopathy may be sufficient.

Supporting tendon excision are the histopathologic findings originally described by Trevino and colleagues[22] and most recently described and reviewed by Mosier and colleagues[23,24] for patients with stage 2 PTT dysfunction as compared with presumably normal cadaver PTTs. In the latter studies, the PTT dysfunction tendons were all enlarged or bulbous with loss of normal color and sheen, giving them a dull white appearance. On microscopic examination there was no evidence of acute or chronic inflammation but instead degenerative tendinosis with a nonspecific reparative response characterized by mucinous degeneration, fibroblast hypercellularity, chondroid metaplasia, and neovascularization resulting in marked disruption in collagen bundle structure and orientation. Therefore, even after debridement a retained PTT will likely always be histopathologically abnormal. Furthermore, the residual bulk of the retained often enlarged PTT, especially if combined with the additional bulk of a tendon transfer, may occasionally lead to discomfort secondary to constriction under a tight flexor retinaculum or alternatively, inability to adequately close the tendon sheath possibly leading to discomfort and decreased mobility secondary to scarring between the tendon and subcutaneous tissue. With respect to concerns about residual strength and function, if the proximal tibialis posterior muscle seems healthy and contractile and the more proximal PTT seems normal, consideration can be made toward tenodesing it to the adjacent FDL transfer. Furthermore, if the distal PTT stump tendon is relatively normal, then it may also be anastomosed to the tendon transfer to preserve the pull on the more distal insertions of the PTT on the plantar foot that help support the arch and adduct the foot.

In addition there may be increased residual strength of the transferred muscle and tendon secondary to hypertrophy, as well as compensation for decreased muscle mass by adjunctive procedures including medial displacement calcaneal osteotomy that increase the moment arm of the transferred tendon relative to the subtalar joint axis. In 12 patients with unilateral stage 2 PTT dysfunction, magnetic resonance imaging (MRI) showed that as compared with the asymptomatic leg, there was mean 10.7% atrophy of the tibialis posterior muscle and 17.2% hypertrophy of the FDL muscle.[25] Eight of these patients were reassessed in a subsequent study[26] an average of 14 months after FDL transfer to the navicular, medial displacement calcaneal osteotomy, and in 4 patients, PTT excision. In the 4 patients with retained PTTs, the PTT muscle volume decreased to 23% of the contralateral side and the FDL muscle volume increased to 11% of the contralateral side. In the 4 patients with resected PTTs, the contralateral side FDL muscle volume increased to 44% of the contralateral side.

Supporting tendon retention is the clinical observation that not all histopathologically abnormal tendons are symptomatic. Patients with tendinopathy involving other tendons in the body including the Achilles tendon often do quite well after treatment including physical therapy, extracorporeal shock wave therapy, platelet-rich plasma injections, or surgical debridement despite residual areas of tendon thickness and nodularity. Many patients with stage 2 PTT dysfunction respond to conservative treatment[27] and have minimal if any tenderness over their abnormal residual PTTs. Gould[28] believed that the strength of the PTT was not fully replaceable by a transfer and that tendon transfer is not necessary if collagen replacement is all that is necessary to restore muscle function. Finally, whereas based on the relative muscle strength data generated by Silver and colleagues[18] the muscles most commonly transferred are significantly weaker than the tibialis posterior, the combined strength of the tibialis posterior and either the FDL or FHL exceeds not only that of the peroneus brevis by itself, but also the combined strength of the peroneus brevis and the other principal evertor of the subtalar joint, the peroneus longus.

The author's personal preference is to debride, repair, and/or augment areas of limited tendinosis and tearing in young or active patients and excise similar tendons in more elderly, low demand patients. A persistently symptomatic retained PTT can still be resected at a later date, but a resected PTT cannot be subsequently reinserted in a patient with symptomatic residual functional weakness.

ALTERNATIVES TO TENDON TRANSFER

A dynamic tendon transfer may not be necessary if the patient's symptoms are not associated with pathology in the PTT or if the PTT can be retained with resolution of pain and restoration of function. Patients with a symptomatic adult-acquired flatfoot deformity, a significant spring ligament tear, and a normal PTT on careful exploration can be treated with a spring ligament repair without any additional intervention to the PTT. Similarly, posterior tibial tendinitis secondary to triceps surae contractures with no PTT abnormalities on MRI or, if believed to be necessary intraoperative exploration, may respond to an isolated gastrocnemius recession. Posterior tibial tenosynovitis surrounding an otherwise normal tendon can be treated with tenosynovectomy.[29,30] An acute PTT laceration may undergo primary repair if the ends can be brought together and small partial-thickness tears in an otherwise normal tendon may be repaired. Symptomatic type 2 accessory naviculars are typically surgically treated with fusion of the synchondrosis[31] or a Kidner procedure[32] with excision of the accessory navicular and distal advancement of the PTT if lax. Patients with symptomatic flatfeet but no PTT tenderness or abnormalities on MRI or intraoperative exploration may undergo an arch-restoring procedure such as arthroereisis, osteotomy, or fusion either without surgical intervention to the PTT, or alternatively PTT advancement[33] or shortening[28] should the tendon be believed to be excessively lax.

The Cobb procedure[34] and Young's tenosuspension[35-37] augment the PTT using the anterior tibial tendon. In the Cobb procedure the medial half of the distal anterior tibial tendon is left attached to its normal insertion on the medial cuneiform and first metatarsal base and the proximal end of the graft sutured to the debrided PTT. In the Young's tenosuspension the distal anterior tibial tendon is rerouted through the navicular, maintaining the normal medial cuneiform and first metatarsal base insertion. Neither of these procedures recreates the function of the tibialis posterior muscle, and in the Cobb procedure whereas the transferred anterior tibial tendon provides healthy tendon for structural support, it has no muscle attached. However, both procedures reinforce the plantar naviculocuneiform ligament to resist the naviculocuneiform sag commonly seen in PTT dysfunction. Both procedures also make the anterior tibialis a less effective antagonist to the peroneus longus, thereby also improving arch height by increasing plantarflexion of the first metatarsal, but at the expense of weakening hindfoot inversion.

With recent complete rupture of the PTT Gould[28] noted that several minutes of traction to the proximal tendon end might pull the contracted muscle out to length and allow direct repair. With more chronic ruptures, if traction to the proximal tendon end produced no or minimal stretch or elasticity, he recommended a tendon transfer. However, if traction produced elasticity, then repair was recommended using one of three techniques: a z-lengthening of the PTT could be performed proximal to the medial malleolus to allow direct repair of the distal tendon ends, the distal gap could be bridged using a plantaris or second toe long extensor tendon interposition graft using a Pulvertaft interweave to both ends of the PTT, or the gap could be bridged by the Cobb method using half of the distal anterior tibial tendon. Other investigators have augmented the debrided PTT using an extensor digitorum longus tendon to the fourth toe graft[38] or either GraftJacket or OrthAdapt biografts[39] instead of tendon transfers, or performed an endoscopic gastrocnemius recession, percutaneous medial displacement calcaneal osteotomy, Evans lateral calcaneal lengthening osteotomy, and in some cases a medial column fusion without surgically addressing the pathologic PTT.[40]

TENDON TRANSFERS

In stage 1 and 2 PTT dysfunction, a dynamic tendon transfer should be considered when active hindfoot inversion motion is still desired and the tibialis posterior is absent, is no longer functional, needs to be excised for significant tendinopathy, or despite consideration of the previously described PTT-preserving procedures is not strong enough to adequately perform its function. Whereas there are indications for tendon transfer in stage 3 and 4 PTT dysfunction, this topic is beyond the scope of this article. The FDL is the most common tendon transfer used in the treatment of PTT dysfunction, although the FHL and peroneal tendons have also been used to reconstruct the PTT.

FDL Transfer

There are several advantages of transferring the FDL to the PTT over the other available tendons. The FDL originates from the posterior tibia adjacent to the tibialis posterior and runs anteromedial and then posterolateral to the PTT without any significant intervening structures from above the flexor retinaculum to the navicular tuberosity. Therefore, the same incision that is used to expose the PTT can be used to harvest and transfer the FDL tendon, although if a longer tendon graft is desired either the incision needs to be lengthened or a second plantar incision added. Furthermore, unlike the FHL and peroneal tendons, the FDL transfer does not need to cross the tibial nerve and posterior tibial vessels. The function of the FDL is more expendable than the other available tendons and, as will be further discussed, is usually at least partially preserved because of the FHL and quadratus plantae attachments on the distal FDL tendon stump. The FDL is also in phase with the tibialis posterior during the gait cycle, although it fires for a shorter percentage of stance phase. The peroneus longus fires during stance phase close to the same amount of time as the tibialis posterior, followed in decreasing order by the FHL, the peroneus brevis, and then the FDL. The main disadvantage of using the FDL is that it is the weakest of the potential donor tendons.

FDL Transfer Surgical Technique

With FDL transfer, if indicated, a triceps surae lengthening procedure is performed first. An initial incision is made overlying the PTT from the level of the medial malleolus to the naviculocuneiform joint (**Fig. 1**). The PTT sheath is opened leaving the flexor retinaculum intact. The PTT is carefully inspected visually and by palpation including the deep surface and distal insertion for any tears, tenosynovitis, thickening, nodularity, or discoloration. An accessory navicular, if present, is excised. If there is any suspicion of a more proximal tendon pathologic condition based on preoperative tenderness, MRI, ultrasound, or intraoperative observation including potential tendoscopy up the proximal tendon sheath, then the incision may be extended more proximally with division and subsequent repair of the flexor retinaculum if needed. A decision is then made as to whether or not the PTT will be preserved and whether or not a tendon transfer will be performed. If an FDL tendon transfer is to be performed,

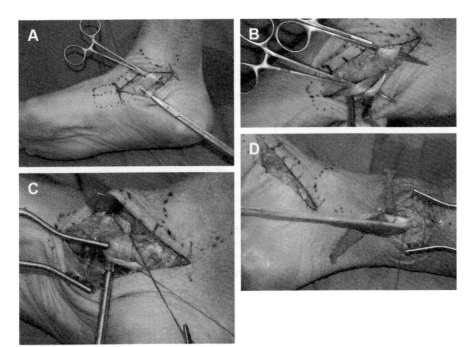

Fig. 1. FDL transfer. (*A*) An incision is made from the naviculocuneiform joint along the PTT to the posterior inferior medial malleolus, which can be extended distally or proximally as needed. The PTT (clamp) and FDL (scissors) are identified in their sheaths. If desired the FDL could be transected here and transferred to the distal PTT in Pulvertaft fashion. (*B*) The incision has been extended distally to the first tarsometatarsal joint level, the abductor hallucis muscle retracted plantarly, and the FDL and if necessary, deeper FHL identified at the master knot of Henry. In this picture the FDL is more superficial and closer to the tip of the clamp than the FHL. (*C*) After making a drill hole in the navicular with an appropriate size reamer over a guide wire, the FDL tendon is passed plantar to dorsal through navicular tunnel and with appropriate tension applied secured with an interference screw to bone and sutures to the distal PTT. (*D*) If the distal PTT has been excised or has ruptured and retracted, the incision is extended proximally or a separate proximal incision made over the tibialis posterior myotendinous junction. The proximal FDL muscle and tendon may be tenodesed to the tibialis posterior muscle and proximal tendon if the latter muscle is functional. If the PTT sheath is healthy-appearing, the distal end of the FDL is brought into the proximal wound and then brought back distally through the PTT sheath under the flexor retinaculum. If not, the FDL tendon is kept in its own sheath. The FDL is then placed through the navicular tunnel and secured as previously described.

the FDL is identified posterolateral to the distal PTT by palpating its tendon sheath while passively flexing and extending the lesser toes. With a knife or dissecting scissor in the FDL sheath deep to the tendon, the sheath is cut distally toward the master knot of Henry, which requires detachment and plantar retraction of the abductor hallucis muscle from the plantar medial aspect of the medial cuneiform, taking care to avoid bleeding vessels that typically cross the field at that level. The medial plantar nerve is often found on the superficial aspect of the FDL tendon,[41] making it important during distal release of the tendon sheath to stay on the deep and not superficial aspect of the FDL tendon. With the ankle plantarflexed, the hindfoot supinated, and the lesser toes plantarflexed, the FDL tendon is carefully transected distally. The length of FDL tendon required depends on where the tendon is being transferred to and the tendon fixation technique used.

Panchbhavi and colleagues[42] described an alternative technique for harvesting the FDL tendon distally through a plantar approach. The FDL tendon sheath was exposed at the level of the medial malleolus and a malleable metal probe with a smooth bulb at the tip introduced into the sheath and passed gently into the midfoot. A separate vertical incision was made through the plantar skin and plantar aponeurosis over the probe and the fibers of the flexor digitorum brevis split to expose the FDL tendon. The location of the plantar incision was found to be typically midway between the base of the heel and the base of the second toe and about two-thirds the width of the foot medially from the lateral border of the foot. After confirming its identity by applying tension to the proximal FDL, the FDL was transected distally and pulled into the proximal wound. In 11 of 83 specimens a slip between the FDL and FHL tendons had to be cut through the distal incision. This connecting slip was exposed by pulling the FDL tendon distally and plantarflexing the hallux in order to pull the FHL tendon distally. There was no injury noted to either the medial or plantar nerve in any of the 83 cadaver specimens, although the medial plantar nerve was noted to be on average 0.7 mm from the FDL division site and the lateral plantar nerve 6.6 mm. Oddy and colleagues[43] compared this limited plantar approach with the traditional medial midfoot exposure and found that the limited plantar approach allowed a mean 22.9 mm additional length of FDL tendon harvest through a mean 15.6 mm decreased incision length.

Some investigators have recommended after harvesting the FDL[44] or FHL[45] tendon for transfer, suturing the distal stump of the tendon to the intact other tendon to maintain plantarflexion strength of the lesser toes or hallux, respectively. Multiple investigators have shown that there are usually, but not always, interconnections between the two tendons near the master knot of Henry.[43,46–50] In one study[49] these interconnections from the FHL to more distal FDL tendon were present in 83 of 95 specimens, with 26 of the 85 specimens having an additional FDL to more distal FHL reciprocal interconnection. In three other studies[46–48] proximal to distal interconnections from the FHL to the FDL were also more common than proximal to distal interconnections from the FDL to FHL, suggesting that preservation of FHL function after transection of the FDL proximal to the master knot of Henry is more likely than preservation of FDL function after transection of the FHL proximal to the master knot of Henry. No interconnections between the FDL and FHL were noted in 4 of 24,[46] 3 of 24,[47] and none of 16[48] specimens. Preoperatively, if the patient can plantarflex the hallux interphalangeal (IP) joint without plantarflexing the lesser toe distal interphalangeal joints, then the surgeon can assume that there is an interconnection from the FHL to the more distal FDL and as long as the FDL tendon is transected proximal to this interconnection at the master knot of Henry, then there should be no need to tenodese the distal stump of the FDL to the FHL. Even if this interconnection is not present, decreased lesser toe distal interphalangeal plantarflexion strength is not functionally limiting for most patients and partially compensated by the quadratus plantae insertion onto the distal FDL and intact metatarsophalangeal and proximal interphalangeal joint plantarflexion from the interossei, lumbricals, and flexor digitorum brevis. Therefore, the author does not extend the midfoot incision distally to perform a tenodesis of the distal FDL stump to the FHL in the absence of this interconnection.

Once harvested, the FDL tendon is stripped of its distal paratenon where it will be placed into bone or tenodesed to tendon or periosteum and a #1 Kessler passing suture placed at the distal end of the tendon. If a decision is made to resect the distal

PTT or if there has been a previous complete rupture with proximal retraction of the tendon, the initial incision is either carried more proximally or a new proximal incision is made over the myotendonous junction of the tibialis posterior and the FDL. If functional and healthy-appearing, the tibialis posterior muscle and proximal-most PTT are tenodesed to the proximal FDL with nonabsorbable suture while physiologic tension is applied to both. Alternatively, this tenodesis can be deferred until later in the procedure after distal fixation of the FDL tendon. If there is not significant scarring in the PTT sheath, particularly under the flexor retinaculum, the FDL tendon is brought into the proximal wound using the passing suture and then rerouted distally through the PTT sheath. If the PTT sheath has significant scarring or adhesions, the FDL tendon is left in its own sheath. If the PTT is being preserved and the FDL tendon is only being transferred to bone or distal tendon, then no exposure of the FDL tendon proximal to the ankle is necessary and the FDL is typically left in its own sheath.

The FDL tendon may be transferred to the navicular, the medial cuneiform, an intact PTT, or should the more proximal tendon require excision, the distal PTT stump. Transferring the FDL tendon into just the distal PTT requires less FDL tendon length and therefore avoids the potential morbidity of a longer midfoot or second plantar incision. Another advantage of transfer directly into the distal PTT or its stump is that it best recreates the normal biomechanical function of the tibialis posterior by acting on all nine bone insertions as opposed to just one. Therefore, even if the FDL is being transferred to the navicular or medial cuneiform, consideration should be given to also tenodesing it to the distal PTT or its stump. Bone fixation of the FDL tendon transfer is required when there is minimal residual distal PTT stump or the distal PTT needs to also be reattached to bone because of partial or complete avulsion, significant laxity, or accessory navicular excision. Biomechanically more secure fixation to bone can also be obtained, which may allow earlier or more aggressive postoperative motion. Of the two bone options, the navicular is the more principal insertion of the PTT and also requires less FDL tendon length to reach it than the medial cuneiform does. However, the theoretical benefit that the FDL transfer to the medial cuneiform provides is it may help support the naviculocuneiform joint, which often develops lateral sag in patients with PTT dysfunction, by buttressing the plantar medial aspect of the joint and by pulling the medial cuneiform plantarly.[12] Mann[44] believed that the placement of the FDL tendon always should be into the navicular bone, not the medial cuneiform because the navicular is positioned more medial to the subtalar joint axis and therefore due to the increased moment arm would be a biomechanically more effective inverter of the subtalar joint and adductor of the foot. A subsequent cadaver study by Hui and colleagues[51] found that transferring the FDL tendon from its native site to the navicular significantly decreased its moment arm 46% and transferring the FDL tendon to the medial cuneiform decreased its moment arm 56%.

Fixation to the distal PTT can be performed using a Pulvertaft weave or a side-to-side repair. The latter may be performed with nonabsorbable suture between the paratenon-free edges of the two tendons or by making a partial-thickness slit in the distal PTT through which debridement can take place and then suture the FDL tendon in the PTT slit like a "hot dog in a bun." When transferred to the navicular or the medial cuneiform, the FDL tendon is typically placed from plantar to dorsal through a bone tunnel that is drilled protecting the proximal and distal articular surfaces and medial cortical wall. In particular, care needs to be taken to avoid violating the concave proximal articular surface of the navicular and damaging the important talonavicular joint. The author will initially place a guide wire through the bone and confirm its position fluoroscopically. A commercially available reamer can then be used over the guide wire to make a tunnel wider than the FDL tendon diameter and appropriate for potential interference screw fixation. A suture passer or thin metal suction tip attached to suction is used to place the passing suture pass through the bone tunnel, which in turn is used to place the FDL tendon into or through the tunnel.

Any pathology noted in the spring ligament is addressed with repair or imbrication with the sutures passed but not yet tied. Adjunctive osteotomies, fusions, or arthroereisis procedures are then performed prior to tying the spring ligament sutures and securing the FDL tendon transfer.

With "appropriate" tension applied to the FDL tendon via the passing suture, the FDL tendon is secured within the navicular or medial cuneiform tunnel using suture anchors,[52,53] interference screws,[54–57] or sewing the distal tendon back to itself. The author finds that typically a plantar to dorsal 15-mm long and 5.5-mm diameter bioabsorbable interference screw in the navicular provides secure fixation for an FDL tendon transected just proximal to the master knot of Henry. The FDL tendon transfer is then further secured by suturing it to the distal PTT and the periosteum at the entrance of the navicular (or medial cuneiform) tunnel, and using a free needle to tie the passing suture to the dorsal navicular (or medial cuneiform) periosteum. If there is inadequate FDL tendon length to reach into the bone tunnel, the FDL tendon may be secured to a plantar bone trough in the navicular or medial cuneiform using a suture anchor and also sutured to the plantar periosteum and distal PTT.

The appropriate tension that the FDL tendon should be secured at is somewhat controversial and principally anecdotal. If the tendon is secured under minimal tension there is concern that the tendon transfer will be weak and nonfunctional. On the other hand, if the tendon is secured in maximum tension there may be concern that there would be limited excursion and decreased function. However, there is some animal evidence that a tendon transfer has at least some ability to adapt to initial overtensioning.[58] There is also the concern that immobilizing the foot in equinus after FDL transfer may lead to residual equinus deformity or diminish the correction after concurrently performed gastrocnemius recession or tendo-Achilles lengthening, thereby increasing long-term biomechanical stress on the FDL tendon transfer. Myerson[59] warned against overtightening the FDL tendon because it might cause subluxation out of the posterior tendon groove. He also recommended performing a tighter repair for heavier patients and those with more extensive deformity and believed that the foot should be positioned beyond the midline and in inversion because it always straightens out and will assume a more neutral position over time. Hansen[60] placed the ankle and forefoot in slight flexion and inversion while pulling the FDL 0.5 to 1.0 cm deep into the medial cuneiform bone, and suturing it over the anterior tibial tendon or dorsal medial cuneiform capsular tissue. Mann[44] firmly pulled on the FDL tendon with the talonavicular joint in full adduction, the subtalar joint in inversion, and the ankle in 20° plantarflexion. Haddad and Mann[16] subsequently recommended securing the FDL tendon transfer at a point halfway between where the tendon sits in the navicular tunnel in its most relaxed state and where it rests when pulled maximally while adducting the transverse tarsal joints and inverting the subtalar joint. Shereff[61] performed his side-to-side anastomosis of the posterior tibial and FDL tendons while holding the foot in plantarflexion and inversion with the toes hyperextended. The author tends to position the foot in 30° to 40° of inversion and 10° to 20° of plantarflexion while tensioning and securing the FDL tendon but usually can still get the ankle to neutral dorsiflexion when splinting at the end of the case.

Whereas there may be a role for the use of biologics with respect to tendon transfer healing to bone and soft tissue as well as subsequent function with respect to gliding in the tendon sheath, the author is not aware of any published data on their use in the surgical treatment of PTT dysfunction.

The posterior tibial and/or FDL tendon sheath(s) are closed distally over the tendon(s) and the flexor retinaculum repaired if disrupted. Care is taken to avoid constricting the tendons with too tight a closure. The incisions are then closed in layers and the leg splinted with the exact position dependent on which adjunct procedures were performed, but ideally in neutral to slight ankle plantarflexion and neutral to slight supination of the hindfoot.

Postoperative rehabilitation is determined by the adjunctive procedures performed and the tendon fixation strength. Isolated FDL transfers may be weight-bearing as tolerated in a cast or boot with protected early motion allowed for reliable patients with secure fixation.

FDL Transfer Results

Goldner and colleagues[50] described using the FDL or FHL for talipes equinovalgus secondary to acute laceration or progressive nontraumatic deformity. They noted that plication of the PTT by itself was insufficient to eliminate pain completely and restore the longitudinal arch and addition of the FDL or FHL tendon transfer improved the result but still was insufficient to produce a pain-free foot with a normal arch. They recommended adding a plication and reinforcement of the medial plantar calcaneonavicular ligament, which they performed along with an Achilles tendon lengthening.

Jahss[62] performed a side-to-side anastomosis of the FDL to an elongated PTT in 6 symptomatic patients with uniformly good results. Inversion strength was restored with an overall 20% to 25% increase in power.

When direct repair of a tear of a short portion of the PTT or reattachment of the distal tendon to the navicular was not possible, Johnson[63] recommended using a proximal and distal side-to-side transfer of the FDL to bridge the gap in the debrided PTT. At 24- to 32-month follow-up all 5 patients who underwent this procedure could do a single-limb heel-rise test and noted considerable subjective improvement with relief of pain in the posteromedial ankle and in the medial arch when weight-bearing, although 3 had continued minor swelling in the region of the medial malleolus.[64]

Mann and Thompson[65] reported on 14 patients who underwent FDL transfer to the navicular and 3 patients who underwent PTT advancement for symptomatic flatfoot deformities. Results were 12 excellent, 1 good, 3 fair, and 1 poor at 2- to 5-year follow-up. The flatfoot deformity was corrected in 4 patients, improved in 7, unchanged in 4, and worse in 2. In a subsequent article Mann[44] stated that the main indication for an FDL transfer was a symptomatic flatfoot deformity secondary to tendinosis of the PTT nonresponsive to conservative treatment with on physical examination at least 15° of subtalar motion, at least 10° of talonavicular adduction, and less than 10° to 12° of fixed forefoot varus. A medial calcaneal osteotomy was added when there was increased calcaneal valgus, or about 80% of the time in his experience. He resected diseased tendon and sutured the proximal PTT to the FDL only in young individuals with isolated areas of tendinosis. Mann also stated that in over a hundred cases in which an isolated FDL transfer was performed for the previously mentioned indications, whereas long-term there seemed to be some minor deterioration of the arch in some cases, fewer than 5% failed and required a subsequent fusion at long-term follow-up. When he did not adhere to the previously mentioned indications, Mann stated the need for revision to a fusion approached 90%.

Conti and colleagues[66] noted that treatment for 6 of 20 patients undergoing isolated PTT debridement and side-to-side anastomosis to the FDL tendon failed at an average of 14.7 months and required subsequent triple arthrodesis.

Shereff[61] reported the results of 17 patients with stage 2 PTT dysfunction who underwent a partial or complete resection of the segment of discolored, attenuated, and damaged tendon followed by end-to-end repair to shorten the PTT and side-to-side tenodesis to the FDL, which was left intact distally. Four of the patients also had a subtalar fusion. At average 27-month follow up all patients had a normal single-limb heel rise and 5/5 inversion strength, all but one patient reported unlimited ambulatory distance, and 10 of the 17 patients displayed an arch nonweightbearing and 7 out of 17 while weightbearing. Of the patients who did not undergo concurrent subtalar fusion, 9 had an excellent American Orthopedic Foot and Ankle society (AOFAS) hindfoot ankle score between 90 and 100, 2 had a good score between 80 and 90, 1 had a fair score between 70 and 80, and 1 patient who was involved in litigation for a motor vehicle accident had a poor score of less than 70.

Gazdag and Cracchiolo[3] resected grossly abnormal areas of the PTT, performed FDL transfers to the navicular, and addressed an associated spring ligament pathologic condition in 17 of 18 patients with stage 2 PTT dysfunction. The 1 patient with a relatively intact PTT underwent tendon shortening and advancement. In an additional 4 patients with stage 2 PTT dysfunction and intact spring ligaments, 3 patients underwent FDL transfers and 1 had a longitudinal split tear repaired. At average 32-month follow-up, 14 of the 18 patients with spring ligament pathology and 2 of the 4 without spring ligament pathology had excellent results with dramatic relief of pain and ability to do a single-leg heel rise, although only 4 had associated active varus angulation of the heel. Two patients with spring ligament pathology and 1 without spring ligament pathology had fair results with mild medial hindfoot pain on exertion and inability to walk more than six blocks, but no limitation of daily activities and the ability to perform a single leg heel rise. The other 3 patients had poor results; 1 who developed reflex sympathetic dystrophy postoperatively, 1 who had medial hindfoot pain that limited daily activities and inability to perform a single-leg heel rise, and 1 with moderate lateral hindfoot pain that limited recreational activities, inability to perform a single-leg heel rise, and mild radiographic talonavicular and subtalar osteoarthritis. The radiographic average lateral talo-first metatarsal angle improved from 13° preoperatively to 9° postoperatively for the 19 patients with excellent or fair results and decreased from 13° to 20° in the 3 patients with poor results, which was because of an increase in 1 of these 3 patients from 12° preoperatively to 32° postoperatively.

Feldman and colleagues[67] performed a similar side-to-side tenodesis of the FDL to the PTT in 11 patients with stage 2 PTT dysfunction. The PTT was debrided, split tears repaired, and in 2 cases of insertional pathologic condition advanced distally on the navicular. At average 34-month follow-up, the mean AOFAS ankle hindfoot score improved from 38.8 preoperatively to 78.1. Five patients had 100% relief of preoperative symptoms, 1 patient had between 90% and 99% relief of preoperative symptoms, 2 patients had between 70% and 89% relief of preoperative symptoms, and 2 patients had poor results with less than 50% pain relief. One of these 2 patients was initially pain-free until her symptoms returned at 18 months postoperatively and the other developed signs consistent with subtalar arthritis at 6 months postoperatively and underwent triple arthrodesis.

Lui[68] described a technique in which PTT debridement and FDL transfer was performed through limited incisions with endoscopic assistance. This procedure was performed along with subtalar arthroereisis and an endoscopically assisted Cobb procedure. One case was illustrated with no residual medial heel or sinus tarsi impingement pain and a well-corrected flatfoot deformity at 21-month follow-up.

FHL Transfer

As noted previously, Goldner and colleagues[50] described using the FDL or FHL for talipes equinovalgus secondary to acute laceration of progressive nontraumatic deformity and added a plication and reinforcement of the medial plantar calcaneo-navicular ligament and Achilles tendon lengthening. Comparing the two transfers, the investigators noted that the FHL was more tendinous than the FDL and had greater muscle mass. They also noted that if left in its normal course under the sustentaculum tali prior to being tightened, sutured to the distal stump of the PTT, and then folded back on itself, the FHL tendon had an excellent stabilizing anchor such that it elevated the sustentaculum tali and aided in relocating the talus.

Sammarco and Hockenberry[45] reported their results for FHL transfer in 17 patients with stage 2 PTT dysfunction. PTT tears were debrided or repaired and a medial displacement calcaneal osteotomy was also performed. The spring ligament was not imbricated or repaired. The FHL tendon was transected at the master knot of Henry and the tendon stump brought proximal to the ankle. The FHL tendon was then passed deep to the tibial nerve and posterior tibial vessels, brought through the PTT sheath, and then sutured to the distal PTT and navicular periosteum. At average 18-month follow-up, the average AOFAS hindfoot score had improved from 62.4 to 83.6. Ten patients were satisfied without reservations, 6 patients were satisfied with minor reservations, and only 1 patient was dissatisfied. There was no statistically significant radiographic or clinical improvement in the longitudinal arch, with only 3 patients having a normal arch and 6 patients with an arch symmetric to the contralateral side.

Several studies have looked at morbidity after principally single incision FHL transfers for Achilles tendinopathy. Richardson and colleagues[69] noted decreased hallux IP plantarflexion strength and decreased pedobarographic pressure under the hallux distal phalanx but normal pressures underneath the first and second metatarsal heads and high scores on the AOFAS Hallux MTP-IP Scale. Coull and colleagues[70] did not notice any functional weakness of the hallux during activities of daily living. Den Hartog[71] also did not note any significant functional deficit or deformity of the hallux. Mulier and colleagues[47] harvested 24 cadaver FHL tendons through a two-incision approach and noted 2 complete ruptures of the medial plantar nerve, 1 partial rupture of both the medial and lateral plantar nerves, and stretching of 3 medial plantar nerves and 1 lateral plantar nerve.

FHL Transfer Surgical Technique

The FHL transfer procedure is done through a similar incision and using many of the same steps as an FDL transfer. The FDL tendon is exposed through the medial midfoot incision to where it crosses superficial to the FHL tendon at the master knot of Henry. The FHL tendon is then identified and with the ankle plantarflexed, the hindfoot supinated, and the hallux IP joint plantarflexed, carefully transected distally (**Fig. 2**). If the patient could preoperatively plantarflex the lesser distal interphalangeal joints without the hallux IP joints simultaneously plantarflexing, suggesting no interconnecting slip from the FDL to the FHL tendon, then consideration could be made for suturing the distal stump of the FHL to the adjacent FDL prior to transecting the FHL tendon. However, if this step is not performed, the resultant usually mild functional loss is typically well-tolerated. The FHL tendon is identified proximal to the flexor retinaculum and the distal FHL tendon stump brought into the proximal wound.

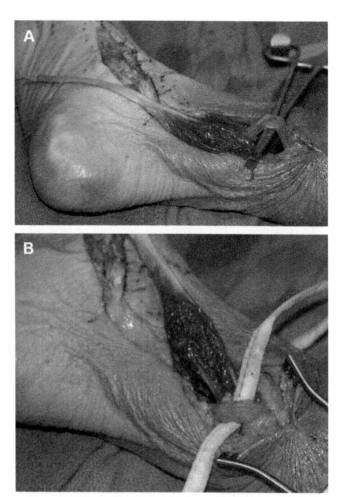

Fig. 2. FHL transfer. The PTT is exposed and debrided through the previously described medial incision(s) (see **Fig. 1**). The FHL tendon is identified and transected at the master knot of Henry and a passing suture placed. (*A*) The distal end of the FHL transfer is then brought into the proximal wound at the level of the tibialis posterior myotendinous junction where it is noted to be posteromedial to the tibial nerve and posterior tibial vessels (clamp). (*B*) The FHL tendon is brought deep and then anterolateral to the neurovascular bundle (ribbon) where it may be tenodesed to healthy tibialis posterior muscle and proximal tendon. The FHL tendon is brought distally through PTT sheath under the flexor retinaculum (see **Fig. 3**B), where it can be placed through a navicular tunnel and then secured to the distal PTT stump as previously described for the flexor digitorum longus transfer already performed in this specimen (see **Fig. 1**).

The tendon is then passed deep to the tibial nerve and posterior tibial vessels, brought through the PTT sheath, and then transferred to the navicular, the medial cuneiform, or the distal PTT similar to an FDL transfer. If the distal PTT is no longer present and the more proximal muscle functional, the proximal tibialis posterior muscle and tendon can be tenodesed to the proximal FHL muscle and tendon similar to how it is performed for an FDL transfer.

Peroneal Tendon Transfers

Song and Deland[72] added a transfer of the peroneus brevis to an FDL transfer, medial displacement calcaneal osteotomy, and if necessary, spring ligament repair for patients with stage 2 PTT dysfunction. The rationale behind the procedure was to provide additional inversion strength to replace the PTT and remove its principal antagonist so that less strength would be required to maintain the arch and invert the subtalar joint. The peroneus brevis transfer was used when the FDL tendon was smaller than usual, which was in less than 10% of cases during the course of their study. The investigators excised the diseased PTT after proximal tenodesis to the FDL. The distal FDL was passed through a drill hole made in the navicular. The peroneus brevis was exposed and released from its insertion from an incision made over the base of the fifth metatarsal, and then brought into a second incision made over the peroneus brevis tendon above the level of the ankle. The tendon was then passed behind the tibia into the proximal medial wound, passed down the PTT sheath, and then placed into the same navicular bony tunnel as the FDL transfer. With the foot held in moderate inversion and plantar flexion both the FDL and peroneus tendons were sewn down to periosteum and soft tissues with nonabsorbable sutures.

For 13 patients with average 20.6-month follow-up there was statistically significant weakness of both hindfoot inversion and eversion as compared with the contralateral unaffected side, although only 1 patient had less than 4/5 hindfoot inversion strength. When retrospectively compared with a matched group of patients of similar age and follow-up that underwent the same procedure without the peroneus brevis transfer, the peroneus brevis group had a nonstatistically significant higher average AOFAS hindfoot score (75.8 vs 71.5) and nonstatistically significant lower average grades of eversion and inversion strength, and eversion range of motion. The investigators stated that subsequent to their study they now only use the peroneus brevis transfer in revision surgery when the FDL is either damaged or no longer available.

Mizel and colleagues[73] reported that 10 patients with no peroneal tendon function secondary to traumatic common peroneal palsy did not develop a hindfoot valgus deformity after transfer of the entire PTT to the dorsal midfoot or one-half the PTT to the peroneus longus at average 75-month follow-up. This article suggests that procedures that decrease peroneus brevis mediated hindfoot eversion and midfoot abduction force would theoretically limit further flatfoot progression and require the repaired or substitute PTT to generate less force to perform its normal function.

Analogous to transferring the peroneus longus to the peroneus brevis in the treatment of the cavus foot,[74] transfer of the peroneus brevis to the peroneus longus would be a logical choice in the treatment of the symptomatic flatfoot, converting deforming abduction force on the fifth metatarsal to arch-correcting plantarflexion force on the first metatarsal. Hansen[75] described a technique that could be performed through the same incision as a lateral column lengthening procedure in which the peroneus brevis was transected at the level of the distal calcaneus, allowed to retract1 to 2 cm, and after removal of its distal paratenon placed through a slit in the peroneus longus with minimal tension and sutured. Hansen also described an alternative technique whereby the peroneus brevis is transected proximal to the superior peroneal retinaculum with the proximal stump placed through a slit in the peroneus longus at physiologic tension. With the foot and ankle held in a neutral plantigrade position, the distal stump of the peroneus brevis is either placed through a more distal slit in the peroneus longus or tenodesed to the distal fibula. No clinical results were given. Schweinberger and Roukis[76] also described their technique for peroneus brevis to peroneus longus transfer along with triceps surae lengthening in diabetic patients undergoing transmetatarsal amputation including the fifth metatarsal base in order to reduce residual midfoot supination and the risk of plantar lateral stump ulceration.

Proximal fractional or z-lengthening of the peroneus brevis would have theoretical benefits in the treatment of stage 2 PTT dysfunction by weakening the PTT's principal antagonist. However, there are also potential negative effects including discomfort secondary to potential subsequent peroneal tendinopathy, functional loss due to weakness of hindfoot eversion, and increased risk of lateral ankle sprain leading to chronic lateral ankle functional instability. Whereas the author has no personal experience with peroneus brevis lengthening or transfer to the peroneus longus in the treatment of PTT dysfunction, the author has had to occasionally perform a complete peroneus brevis tenotomy along with a triceps surae lengthening procedure in order to realign a significant stage 3 PTT dysfunction deformity during triple arthrodesis.

Whereas the peroneus longus tendon is also an antagonist to the PTT in the sense that it is a strong evertor of the hindfoot, it also helps maintain the longitudinal arch of the foot by plantarflexing the first metatarsal and supporting the plantar ligaments of the midfoot, particularly the first tarsometatarsal joint. Fried and Hendel[77] described transferring the peroneus longus, as well as the FDL, FHL, and extensor hallucis longus tendons, to the paralyzed PTTs of children with calcaneovalgus deformities secondary to poliomyelitis. However, the author is not aware of any published descriptions of transferring the peroneus longus to the PTT in the treatment of adult PTT dysfunction, although it has been used clinically to reconstruct the spring ligament.[5]

Peroneus Brevis Tendon Transfer Surgical Technique

The peroneus brevis tendon transfer procedure is also done using the same medial incision(s) and many of the same steps as a PTT debridement and FDL transfer. In addition, incisions are made over the course of the peroneus brevis tendon just proximal to the fifth metatarsal base insertion and posterior to the fibula at the level of the tibialis posterior myotendinous junction. The peroneus brevis is identified and transected distally. With the aid of a passing suture and a long curved clamp, the peroneus brevis tendon is then brought into the proximal lateral incision (**Fig. 3**). The peroneus brevis tendon and some of its attached muscle is then passed deep to the peroneus longus, FHL, tibial nerve, and posterior tibial vessels into the proximal medial incision. The peroneus brevis may then be tenodesed to the proximal tibialis posterior muscle, brought through the distal PTT sheath, and then transferred to the navicular, medial cuneiform, or distal PTT similar to or in addition to an FDL transfer.

ROLE OF ISOLATED SOFT TISSUE PROCEDURES IN STAGE 2 PTT DYSFUNCTION

It is current orthopedic dogma that patients with stage 2 PTT dysfunction for whom appropriate nonoperative treatment fails require more than just soft tissue procedures addressing the PTT pathology with tendon debridement and repair, advancement, or transfer; spring and/or deltoid ligament pathology; and significant triceps surae contractures. The addition of concurrent arch-improving procedures has been strongly recommended including arthroereisis, osteotomy, and fusion of joints not considered critical for normal hindfoot function.

However, whereas these additional bone procedures seem to be associated in the orthopedic literature with overall good short- and intermediate-term results including improved radiographic correction as compared with isolated soft tissue procedures, they are not without added morbidity. Fusions and osteotomies may require

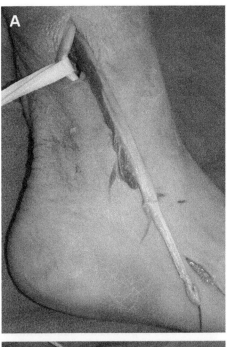

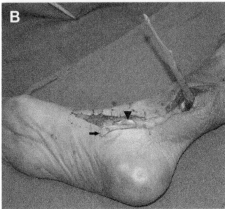

Fig. 3. Peroneus brevis transfer. The PTT is exposed and debrided through the previously described medial incision(s) (see **Fig. 1**). (*A*) The peroneus brevis tendon is identified through two lateral incisions, one made just proximal to the fifth metatarsal base insertion and the other posterior to the fibula at the level of the tibialis posterior myotendinous junction. The peroneus brevis is transected distally and brought into the proximal lateral incision with the aid of a passing suture. The peroneus brevis is identified deep to the more superficial peroneus longus tendon (ribbon). (*B*) Using a clamp deep to the tibial nerve, posterior tibial vessels, and flexor hallucis longus, the peroneus brevis is kept deep to the peroneus longus and passed from the proximal lateral incision into the proximal medial incision where it may be tenodesed to the tibialis posterior at the level of its myotendinous junction. The peroneus brevis is then brought distally through the PTT sheath under the flexor retinaculum, similar to how the flexor hallucis longus (*arrow*) was previously passed in this specimen for **Fig. 2** The peroneus brevis can then be placed through a navicular tunnel and secured to the distal PTT as previously performed for the flexor digitorum longus tendon (*arrowhead*) in this specimen for **Fig. 1**.

prolonged nonweightbearing immobilization, which may be particularly difficult for elderly patients or those with a symptomatic contralateral lower extremity pathology. There may be symptomatic malunion, nonunion, undercorrection, overcorrection, or hardware that requires additional surgery. Although typically there is increased arch improvement, not uncommonly there is still residual planovalgus deformity, sometimes significant, particularly if only one osteotomy was performed for a severe preoperative deformity. Some patients who have had significant flatfoot deformities all their life find suddenly having a normal arch, particularly one that is unilateral, difficult to get used to and feel as if they are walking on the lateral aspect of their foot. There are people with nonweightbearing cavovarus feet who have developed symptomatic weightbearing planovalgus deformities over time. The author has seen medial displacement calcaneal osteotomy in conjunction with other procedures including spring ligament repair and FDL transfer in these people lead to significant postoperative hindfoot varus with subsequent symptomatic development of lateral foot pain and/or lateral ankle stability. Evans calcaneal osteotomy may be associated with symptomatic bone impingement in the sinus tarsi and increased forefoot supination. If not addressed, this forefoot varus/supination may drive the hindfoot back into valgus analogous to the cavovarus foot where forefoot valgus secondary to a plantarflexed first metatarsal can cause compensatory hindfoot varus. Sural incisional neuromas may develop after medial displacement calcaneal osteotomy. Arthroereisis components not uncommonly need to be removed secondary to lateral subtalar irritation and the long-term effects of particulate debris from metal, polylactic acid, and more historically silicone and polyethylene on the adjacent bone and articular surfaces of the posterior facet are unknown.

Given the previously described morbidity and the fairly good short-term results for most of the previously discussed reports describing isolated soft tissue procedures including tendon transfer in stage 2 PTT dysfunction,[3,44,50,61,62,64–67] it may be reasonable to consider performing isolated soft tissue procedures in patients with mild stage 2 deformity or elderly low demand patients with mild to moderate deformity. Many of these patients will do quite well with PTT debridement, repair, and/or transfer, spring ligament imbrication or repair, and if needed, gastrocnemius recession. A minority of these patients will have noticeable improvement in their arch. Many of the rest may tolerate residual planovalgus deformity, which in many cases they have done for most of their life including their contralateral foot. Furthermore, the medial soft tissue repair may be biomechanically protected by postoperative use of an insole orthosis and once adequate soft tissue healing has occurred, an aggressive therapy program similar to those often used successfully in the nonoperative treatment of stage 2 PTT dysfunction.[27] The patients may be early weightbearing as tolerated in a cast or boot, which may avoid placement in an extended care facility for an elderly patient with bilateral PTT dysfunction or symptomatic contralateral extremity arthritis.

In the study with the overall worst reported results for isolated soft tissue procedures,[66] 30% of the 20 patients had a failure of their reconstruction and required subsequent triple arthrodesis. However, 70% of the patients did not and may have avoided an initial triple arthrodesis with less residual postoperative motion and function. Also in that particular study, treatment for only 1 of 8 patients with grade I tears of their PTT by preoperative MRI failed and required triple arthrodesis.

Furthermore, if an isolated soft tissue procedure is unsuccessful, minimal bridges have burned and a more extensive bone procedure can subsequently be added. If the medial soft tissue procedure has failed, a tendon transfer can be performed if not done originally; the previous tendon transfer may undergo debridement, advancement, or replacement transfer with the remaining FDL, FHL, or peroneus brevis tendons, or biografts,[39] or a hindfoot fusion performed. Therefore, whereas the author would still recommend considering adjunctive bone procedures for most patients undergoing surgery for stage 2 PTT dysfunction, particularly those patients who are younger, more active, or who have more significant deformities, there are several situations where with appropriate patient counseling about expectations the author believes an isolated soft tissue procedure that may include tendon transfer is quite reasonable.

REFERENCES

1. Johnson KA, Strom DE. Tibialis posterior tendon dysfunction. Clin Orthop Relat Res 1989;(239):196–206.
2. Myerson MS. Adult acquired flatfoot deformity: treatment of dysfunction of the posterior tibial tendon. Instr Course Lect 1997;46:393–405.
3. Gazdag AR, Cracchiolo A 3rd. Rupture of the posterior tibial tendon. Evaluation of injury of the spring ligament and clinical assessment of tendon transfer and ligament repair. J Bone Joint Surg Am 1997;79(5):675–81.
4. Jeng CL, Bluman EM, Myerson MS. Minimally invasive deltoid ligament reconstruction for stage IV flatfoot deformity. Foot Ankle Int 2011;32(1):21–30.
5. Williams BR, Ellis SJ, Deyer TW, et al. Reconstruction of the spring ligament using a peroneus longus autograft tendon transfer. Foot Ankle Int 2010;31(7):567–77.
6. Aronow MS. Triceps surae contractures associated with posterior tibial tendon dysfunction. Tech Orthop 2000;15:164–73.
7. Needleman RL. A surgical approach for flexible flatfeet in adults including a subtalar arthroereisis with the MBA sinus tarsi implant. Foot Ankle Int 2006;27(1):9–18.
8. Guyton GP, Jeng C, Krieger LE, et al. Flexor digitorum longus transfer and medial displacement calcaneal osteotomy for posterior tibial tendon dysfunction: a middle-term clinical follow-up. Foot Ankle Int 2001;22(8):627–32.
9. Myerson MS, Badekas A, Schon LC. Treatment of stage II posterior tibial tendon deficiency with flexor digitorum longus tendon transfer and calcaneal osteotomy. Foot Ankle Int 2004;25(7):445–50.
10. Thomas RL, Wells BC, Garrison RL, et al. Preliminary results comparing two methods of lateral column lengthening. Foot Ankle Int 2001;22(2):107–19.
11. Hirose CB, Johnson JE. Plantar flexion opening wedge medial cuneiform osteotomy for correction of fixed forefoot varus associated with flatfoot deformity. Foot Ankle Int 2004;25(8):568–74.
12. Moseir-LaClair S, Pomeroy G, Manoli A 2nd. Intermediate follow-up on the double osteotomy and tendon transfer procedure for stage II posterior tibial tendon insufficiency. Foot Ankle Int 2001;22(4):283–91.
13. Toolan BC, Sangeorzan BJ, Hansen ST Jr. Complex reconstruction for the treatment of dorsolateral peritalar subluxation of the foot. Early results after distraction arthrodesis of the calcaneocuboid joint in conjunction with stabilization of, and transfer of the flexor digitorum longus tendon to, the midfoot to treat acquired pes planovalgus in adults. J Bone Joint Surg Am 1999;81(11):1545–60.
14. Chi TD, Toolan BC, Sangeorzan BJ, et al. The lateral column lengthening and medial column stabilization procedures. Clin Orthop Relat Res 1999;(365):81–90.
15. Johnson JE, Cohen BE, DiGiovanni BF, et al. Subtalar arthrodesis with flexor digitorum longus transfer and spring ligament repair for treatment of posterior tibial tendon insufficiency. Foot Ankle Int 2000;21(9):722–9.

16. Haddad SL, Mann RA. Flatfoot in adults. In: Coughlin MJ, Mann RA, Saltzman C, editors. Surgery of the foot and ankle. 8th edition. St Louis (MO): Mosby; 2011. p. 1007–86.

17. Bluman EM, Dowd T. The basics and science of tendon transfers. Foot Ankle Clin 2011;16(3):385–99.

18. Silver RL, de la Garza J, Rang M. The myth of muscle balance. A study of relative strengths and excursions of normal muscles about the foot and ankle. J Bone Joint Surg Br 1985;67(3):432–7.

19. Kitaoka HB, Luo ZP, An KN. Subtalar arthrodesis versus flexor digitorum longus tendon transfer for severe flatfoot deformity: an in vitro biomechanical analysis. Foot Ankle Int 1997;18(11):710–5.

20. Kitaoka HB, Luo ZP, An KN. Reconstruction operations for acquired flatfoot: biomechanical evaluation. Foot Ankle Int 1998;19(4):203–7.

21. Arangio GA, Salathe EP. A biomechanical analysis of posterior tibial tendon dysfunction, medial displacement calcaneal osteotomy and flexor digitorum longus transfer in adult acquired flat foot. Clin Biomech (Bristol, Avon) 2009;24(4):385–90.

22. Trevino S, Gould N, Korson R. Surgical treatment of stenosing tenosynovitis at the ankle. Foot Ankle 1981;2(1):37–45.

23. Mosier SM, Lucas DR, Pomeroy G, et al. Pathology of the posterior tibial tendon in posterior tibial tendon insufficiency. Foot Ankle Int 1998;19(8):520–4.

24. Mosier SM, Pomeroy G, Manoli A 2nd. Pathoanatomy and etiology of posterior tibial tendon dysfunction. Clin Orthop Relat Res 1999;(365):12–22.

25. Wacker J, Calder JD, Engstrom CM, et al. MR morphometry of posterior tibialis muscle in adult acquired flat foot. Foot Ankle Int 2003;24(4):354–7.

26. Rosenfeld PF, Dick J, Saxby TS. The response of the flexor digitorum longus and posterior tibial muscles to tendon transfer and calcaneal osteotomy for stage II posterior tibial tendon dysfunction. Foot Ankle Int 2005;26(9):671–4.

27. Alvarez RG, Marini A, Schmitt C, et al. Stage I and II posterior tibial tendon dysfunction treated by a structured nonoperative management protocol: an orthosis and exercise program. Foot Ankle Int 2006;27(1):2–8.

28. Gould JS. Direct repair of the posterior tibial tendon. Foot Ankle Clin 1997;2(2): 275–80.

29. Bare AA, Haddad SL. Tenosynovitis of the posterior tibial tendon. Foot Ankle Clin 2001;6(1):37–66.

30. Teasdall RD, Johnson KA. Surgical treatment of stage I posterior tibial tendon dysfunction. Foot Ankle Int 1994;15(12):646–8.

31. Malicky ES, Levine DS, Sangeorzan BJ. Modification of the Kidner procedure with fusion of the primary and accessory navicular bones. Foot Ankle Int 1999;20(1):53–4.

32. Kidner FC. The pre-hallux (accessory scaphoid) and its relation to flatfoot. J Bone Joint Surg 1929;11(4):831–7.

33. Miller OL. A plastic flat foot operation. J Bone Joint Surg 1927;9(1):84–91.

34. Knupp M, Hintermann B. The Cobb procedure for treatment of acquired flatfoot deformity associated with stage II insufficiency of the posterior tibial tendon. Foot Ankle Int 2007;28(4):416–21.

35. Jacobs AM. Soft tissue procedures for the stabilization of medial arch pathology in the management of flexible flatfoot deformity. Clin Podiatr Med Surg 2007;24(4):657–65, vii–viii.

36. Sekiya JK, Saltzman CL. Long term follow-up of medial column fusion and tibialis anterior transposition for adolescent flatfoot deformity. Iowa Orthop J 1997;17:121–9.

37. Young CS. Operative treatment of pes planus. Surg Gynecol Obstet 1939;99:1099–101.

38. Kettlekamp BB, Alexander HH. Spontaneous rupture of the posterior tibial tendon. J Bone Joint Surg Am 1969;51A(4):759–64.
39. Lee D. Effects of posterior tibial tendon augmented with biografts and calcaneal osteotomy in stage II adult-acquired flatfoot deformity. Foot Ankle Spec 2009;2(1): 27–31.
40. Didomenico L, Stein DY, Wargo-Dorsey M. Treatment of posterior tibial tendon dysfunction without flexor digitorum tendon transfer: a retrospective study of 34 patients. J Foot Ankle Surg 2011;50(3):293–8.
41. Sullivan RJ, Aronow MS. Anatomical relationships of the medial plantar nerve within the midfoot. Presented at the American Orthopaedic Foot and Ankle Society 17th Annual Summer Meeting. San Diego (CA), July 19, 2001.
42. Panchbhavi VK, Yang J, Vallurupalli S. Minimally invasive method of harvesting the flexor digitorum longus tendon: a cadaver study. Foot Ankle Int 2008;29(1):42–8.
43. Oddy MJ, Flowers MJ, Davies MB. Flexor digitorum longus tendon exposure for flatfoot reconstruction: a comparison of two methods in a cadaveric model. Foot Ankle Surg 2010;16(2):87–90.
44. Mann RA. Posterior tibial tendon dysfunction. Treatment by flexor digitorum longus transfer. Foot Ankle Clin 2001;6(1):77–87.
45. Sammarco GJ, Hockenbury RT. Treatment of stage II posterior tibial tendon dysfunction with flexor hallucis longus transfer and medial displacement calcaneal osteotomy. Foot Ankle Int 2001;22(4):305–12.
46. LaRue BG, Anctil EP. Distal anatomical relationship of the flexor hallucis longus and flexor digitorum longus tendons. Foot Ankle Int 2006;27(7):528–32.
47. Mulier T, Rummens E, Dereymaeker G. Risk of neurovascular injuries in flexor hallucis longus tendon transfers: an anatomic cadaver study. Foot Ankle Int 2007;28(8): 910–5.
48. O'Sullivan E, Carare-Nnadi R, Greenslade J, et al. Clinical significance of variations in the interconnections between flexor digitorum longus and flexor hallucis longus in the region of the knot of Henry. Clin Anat 2005;18(2):121–5.
49. Wapner KL, Hecht PJ, Shea JR, et al. Anatomy of second muscular layer of the foot: considerations for tendon selection in transfer for Achilles and posterior tibial tendon reconstruction. Foot Ankle Int 1994;15(8):420–3.
50. Goldner JL, Keats PK, Bassett FH 3rd, et al. Progressive talipes equinovalgus due to trauma or degeneration of the posterior tibial tendon and medial plantar ligaments. Orthop Clin North Am 1974;5(1):39–51.
51. Hui HE, Beals TC, Brown NA. Influence of tendon transfer site on moment arms of the flexor digitorum longus muscle. Foot Ankle Int 2007;28(4):441–7.
52. Myerson MS, Cohen I, Uribe J. An easy way of tensioning and securing a tendon to bone. Foot Ankle Int 2002;23(8):753–5.
53. Sullivan RJ, Gladwell HA, Aronow MS, et al. An in vitro study comparing the use of suture anchors and drill hole fixation for flexor digitorum longus transfer to the navicular. Foot Ankle Int 2006;27(5):363–6.
54. Harris NJ, Ven A, Lavalette D. Flexor digitorum longus transfer using an interference screw for stage 2 posterior tibial tendon dysfunction. Foot Ankle Int 2005;26(9): 781–2.
55. Louden KW, Ambrose CG, Beaty SG, et al. Tendon transfer fixation in the foot and ankle: a biomechanical study evaluating two sizes of pilot holes for bioabsorbable screws. Foot Ankle Int 2003;24(1):67–72.
56. Sabonghy EP, Wood RM, Ambrose CG, et al. Tendon transfer fixation: comparing a tendon to tendon technique vs. bioabsorbable interference-fit screw fixation. Foot Ankle Int 2003;24(3):260–2.

57. Wukich DK, Rhim B, Lowery NJ, et al. Biotenodesis screw for fixation of FDL transfer in the treatment of adult acquired flatfoot deformity. Foot Ankle Int 2008;29(7):730–4.
58. Takahashi M, Ward SR, Marchuk LL, et al. Asynchronous muscle and tendon adaptation after surgical tensioning procedures. J Bone Joint Surg Am 2010;92(3):664–74.
59. Myerson MS. Correction of flatfoot deformity in the adult. In: Myerson MS, Reconstructive foot and ankle surgery. Philadelphia: Elsevier Saunders; 2005. p. 189–215.
60. Hansen ST. Transfer of the flexor digitorum communis to the first cuneiform. In: Hansen ST. Functional reconstruction of the foot and ankle. Philadelphia: Lippincott, Williams & Wilkins; 2000. p. 430–2.
61. Shereff, MJ. Treatment of the ruptured posterior tibial tendon with direct repair and tenodesis. Foot Ankle Clin 1997;2(2):281–96.
62. Jahss MH. Spontaneous rupture of the tibialis posterior tendon: clinical findings, tenographic studies, and a new technique of repair. Foot Ankle 1982;3(3):158–66.
63. Johnson KA. Tibialis posterior tendon rupture. Clin Orthop Relat Res 1983;(177):140–7.
64. Funk DA, Cass JR, Johnson KA. Acquired adult flat foot secondary to posterior tibial-tendon pathology. J Bone Joint Surg Am 1986;68(1):95–102.
65. Mann RA, Thompson FM. Rupture of the posterior tibial tendon causing flat foot. Surgical treatment. J Bone Joint Surg Am 1985;67(4):556–61.
66. Conti S, Michelson J, Jahss M. Clinical significance of magnetic resonance imaging in preoperative planning for reconstruction of posterior tibial tendon ruptures. Foot Ankle 1992;13(4):208–14.
67. Feldman NJ, Oloff LM, Schulhofer SD. In situ tibialis posterior to flexor digitorum longus tendon transfer for tibialis posterior tendon dysfunction: a simplified surgical approach with outcome of 11 patients. J Foot Ankle Surg 2001;40(1):2–7.
68. Lui TH. Endoscopic assisted posterior tibial tendon reconstruction for stage 2 posterior tibial tendon insufficiency. Knee Surg Sports Traumatol Arthrosc 2007;15(10):1228–34.
69. Richardson DR, Willers J, Cohen BE, et al. Evaluation of the hallux morbidity of single-incision flexor hallucis longus tendon transfer. Foot Ankle Int 2009;30(7):627–30.
70. Coull R, Flavin R, Stephens MM. Flexor hallucis longus tendon transfer: evaluation of postoperative morbidity. Foot Ankle Int 2003;24(12):931–4.
71. Den Hartog BD. Flexor hallucis longus transfer for chronic Achilles tendonosis. Foot Ankle Int 2003;24(3):233–7.
72. Song SJ, Deland JT. Outcome following addition of peroneus brevis tendon transfer to treatment of acquired posterior tibial tendon insufficiency. Foot Ankle Int 2001;22(4):301–4.
73. Mizel MS, Temple HT, Scranton PE Jr, et al. Role of the peroneal tendons in the production of the deformed foot with posterior tibial tendon deficiency. Foot Ankle Int 1999;20(5):285–9.
74. Ryssman DB, Myerson MS. Tendon transfers for the adult flexible cavovarus foot. Foot Ankle Clin 2011;16(3):435–50.
75. Hansen ST. Transfer of the peroneus brevis to the peroneus longus. In: Hansen ST. Functional reconstruction of the foot and ankle. Philadelphia: Lippincott, Williams & Wilkins; 2000. p. 439–41.
76. Schweinberger MH, Roukis TS. Balancing of the transmetatarsal amputation with peroneus brevis to peroneus longus tendon transfer. J Foot Ankle Surg 2007;46(6):510–4.
77. Fried A, Hendel C. Paralytic deformity of the ankle: replacement of the paralyzed tibialis posterior by the peronaeus longus. J Bone Joint Surg Am 1959;39A(4):921–32.

Young's Procedure for the Treatment of Valgus Flatfoot Deformity Caused by a Posterior Tibial Tendon Dysfunction, Stage II

Nuri Schinca, MD[a],*, Alicia Lasalle, MD[b], Josefina Alvarez, MD[a]

KEYWORDS

- Flatfoot • Supple flatfoot • Tendon translocation
- Tibialis posterior tendon insufficiency

KEY POINTS

- Young's procedure achieves a good muscle balance.
- The tibial anterior tendon is not detached therefore, it works actively.
- The technique improves the medial arch providing it with active components.
- It causes an insufficiency of the ATT, which results in a predominance of the peroneus longus.
- It reinforces soft parts of the plantar and medial sector.
- It does not sacrifice the joint mobility.

Flatfoot in adults caused by a dysfunction of the posterior tibial tendon is a frequent pathology for which several therapies have been proposed, for instance tendon transfers and bone procedures.

In Uruguay, in 1974, Dr Selva Ruiz and Professor Dr Liber Mauro[1] began to use the procedure described by Young[2] to treat supple flatfoot in children and adolescents, because they understood it contained an action mechanism that worked better than other techniques on the pathophysiology of the deformity. This technique consisted of the translocation of the tendon from the tibial anterior muscle, changing its route by means of a tunnel carved in the navicular.

Even when the use of flexors is advised all over the world for the treatment of adult flatfoot[3] caused by a posterior tibial tendon (PTT) dysfunction, in view of the good

[a] Foot and Ankle Surgery Service, British Hospital, Italia Avenue 2420, CP 11600, Montevideo, Uruguay; [b] Foot and Ankle Surgery Service, Police Hospital, José Batlle y Ordoñez 3574, CP 11700, Montevideo, Uruguay
* Corresponding author. San Salvador 2274/301. CP 11200, Montevideo, Uruguay.
E-mail address: florin@chasque.net

Foot Ankle Clin N Am 17 (2012) 227–245
doi:10.1016/j.fcl.2012.02.002
1083-7515/12/$ – see front matter © 2012 Elsevier Inc. All rights reserved.

results obtained with Young's procedure in supple flatfoot deformity (FFD) of children and adolescents, and considering that it was a technique we were familiarized with, we decided to use it also for the treatment of FFD caused by PTT dysfunction in adults.

PATHOPHYSIOLOGY

Navarro[4] claimed that the study of the anatomy alone is not enough to understand the modifications that characterize the lesions or illnesses, "as the pathology does not only alter the form or structure, but it also affects the function." Understanding the anatomy of the foot allows us to comprehend how the foot adapted itself to the changes necessary for humans to stand and walk.

Among those changes, the medial arch was shaped, which is characteristic of human beings and represents a static platform in the foot support and a propulsion lever in its dynamic function. Mauro[5] states that the dome is structured by arches. These are true springs constituted by juxtaposed bone pieces, supported by capsule–ligament systems. The main support areas are eccentric: The calcaneus on the back, and metatarsal heads and toes on the front. This submits the columns to tensile and compressive forces. The compressive forces follow the trabecular bone systems, the tensile forces are resisted by the plantar capsule–ligament systems, which constitute powerful tensors.

From a pathophysiologic point of view, we consider the foot as constituted of 4 links, 3 peripheral and 1 central (the talus). The peripheral links are active, that is to say, they are subject to the influence of forces capable of unbalancing the foot. These forces are represented by gravity and/or muscle driving forces.

1. The upper link is constituted by the tibial plafond and the ankle mortise, and it is through.
2. This link that the pressure forces arrive. The mortise is not rigid, owing to the inferior tibiofibular joint. The lateral malleolus is an external stabilizer of the hind foot, it is stronger and more posterior, and it descends further than the medial malleolus.
3. The single posterior link is represented by the calcaneus, preceded in its dynamics by a sole motor: The powerful triceps surae.
4. The anterior link, with a more complex structure, multisegmental, is constituted by the pre talus foot.
5. The central link is represented by the talus. This bone has key characteristics:
   a. It constitutes the central organ of the hind foot.
   b. It is intra-articular, surrounded by wide cartilaginous surfaces.
   c. It resembles a "patella" bone: embedded in the malleolar pincer, it receives and distributes the forces transmitted by the tibia towards the plantar architecture.
   d. It is a bone "relais" of the 2 ligament chains that originate in the malleoli[6]; therefore, its stability is ensured by the fact that it is embedded and the richness of the ligament insertions.
   e. It is a passive link in the kinetic chain of the foot, because it does not offer insertion for any muscle.
   f. It is not the leader of any movement. Connected to the 3 peripheral links, it is subjected to their influences.

THE JOINT COMPLEX OF THE HINDFOOT

The center of the hindfoot architecture is the talus. Around it, a ball joint is constituted, the powerful peritalar joint. This joint comprises 3 other articulations, anatomically separated but closely linked from the functional point of view:

1. The tibiofibular talar joint.
2. The posterior subtalar joint.
3. The anterior subtalar and the talonavicular joint, both form a complex structure. The head of talus is embedded in a cotyloid fossa built of bone structures: Glenoid cavity of the navicular and sustentacular facet, all of them structure the coxa pedis.
4. A ligament "coat" constituted by the spring ligament, covered by cartilage and reinforced by the tibialis posterior, and the deltoid ligament or tibionavicular gleno sustentacular ligament. The cavity is completed by the dorsal talonavicular ligament and the Y-ligament. The navicular bone has a "glenoid" reception cavity, wider than the corresponding articular surface of the talus, thus facilitating a broad rotation movement.[4]

At the same time, the talus head is parabolic. This suggests a blocking mechanism with the navicular, capable of reaching a higher position than the calcaneocuboid joint, resulting in the development of the arch. Here is where the PTT takes part, blocking the subtalar joint before the foot is lifted, so that the triceps elevates the heel from the ground. The calcaneus plays an anatomic role on the joint complex of the hindfoot, in its lateral sector, by means of the posterior subtalar joint. However, at the same time, it is closely linked, from the functional point of view, with the anterior sector of the coxa pedis, because its vast tuberosity articulates with the cuboid bone. In this way, even when it belongs to the outer edge of the foot, it constitutes the rotation sector of the hindfoot, together with the joints referred to as "peritalar joint." The muscle systems that control foot mobility are very complex:

1. All the muscles are polyarticular.
2. All of them are inserted distally through the front of the midtarsal joint, with the exception of the triceps surae.
3. They all act on the heterokinetic cardan joint of the hindfoot. Their actions take place in accordance with the flexion-extension and the inversion-eversion movements.
4. According to Kapandji's scheme,[6] the muscle dynamic in relation to the cardan axis allows for the following muscle categorization:
   a. Anterior-external: Dorsiflexors–evertors: Extensor digitorum longus and peroneus brevis;
   b. Posterior-external: Plantar flexors–evertors: Peroneus brevis and longus, which control the foot curvature;
   c. Posterior-internal: Plantar flexors–invertors: Triceps surae, tibialis posterior and flexor digitorum; and
   d. Anterior-internal: Dorsiflexors–supinators: Extensors hallux and tibial anterior.

As we see, there are synergy–antagonism actions. The muscle system of the first metatarsal is constituted by 2 antagonist muscles: The tibialis anterior tendon (ATT) that lifts it and gets it into a horizontal position, determining the supination of the entire forefoot,[5] and the peroneus longus, which is a depressor of the first metatarsal, and abductor and pronator of the forefoot. It depresses the forefoot and moves it outward joining the internal and external metatarsals, superimposing them, facilitating and optimizing the plantar flexion function of the triceps surae.

The unbalance of this couple is among the pathogenic factors of the flatfoot. The main cause of adult flatfoot is the loss of the muscular function. Several pathogenic mechanisms combine causing isolated or combined effects.[7,8] The flatfoot is not only a depression or reduction in height of the anteroposterior dome in standing position, but is a clinical radiologic complex that adds to this remarkable sign, the valgus position of the heel, the emergence of the head of the talus in the inner edge, the retraction of the Achilles tendon, and the abduction and supination of the forefoot.

The injured PTT loses its supportive and cavus action, producing a valgus hindfoot and a flattening of the foot arch. The PTT is no longer able to block the hindfoot in varus to allow the Achilles tendon and the hindfoot to lift the heel, thus becoming unstable. Instead of being transmitted to the anterior and posterior pillars, the forces arriving to the foot are now affecting the conflict and stress area of the inner edge. This results in a progressive elongation and/or rupture of the medial and plantar capsular ligamentous complex, becoming an aggressor to the static of the foot.[9]

The valgus displacement of the calcaneus restrains the main support of the talus, and allows for its inward–forward translocation in plantar flexion, misdirecting the entire peritalar joint: The tibiotalar, subtalar, and midtarsal relation. With the heel bone in pronation, the Achilles tendon will not produce a supinator effect over the hindfoot (as it occurs with a normal foot); instead, because it is inserted in a valgus heel bone, it becomes a pronator.

The triceps has the property of reinforcing the pronation or supination movement, responding to the behavior of the varus or valgus calcaneus. What is more, with time, it retracts, resulting in a hindfoot equinus. Keeping the heel in valgus and the ankle in plantar flexion shortens the tendon and, with time, diminishes the push off or lifting force of the triceps. Delayed heel-off is characteristic of valgus flatfoot stage II.[10–15] The forefoot is displaced in abduction, with the navicular and cuboid located outside the posterior tarsus. A subluxation of the talonavicular joint takes place. Subsequently, the metatarsal shafts may try to compensate by assuming an abduction and supination position, and this breaks the talus–navicular–cuneiform metatarsal axis.

The valgus hindfoot secondarily determines an increase of the pressure under the head of the first metatarsal, which becomes horizontal. The retraction of the tibialis anterior aggravates the situation. With the hindfoot in valgus deviation, the supination is caused by accommodative changes that allow the medial and lateral columns of the forefoot to remain in contact with the ground.[16]

There are authors, like Hintermann and colleagues,[17] who state that the supination attitude of the forefoot appears earlier than the insufficiency of the tibialis posterior, so that in the semiological analysis, this sign appears before the tiptoe sign, which tells of the importance of searching for the first ray elevation sign.

We believe that the first ray elevation sign is secondary to the appearance of the flatfoot deformity. What aspects should be considered by a technique that pretends to correct the valgus flatfoot deformity caused by a PTT dysfunction?

1. Insufficiency of the PTT.
2. Valgus hind foot.
3. Elongation or rupture of the internal capsule–ligament structures.
4. Forefoot supination.
5. Forefoot abduction.

How is it possible to correct this muscle imbalance, caused by the posterior tibialis insufficiency and how is Young's procedure able to achieve it?

TECHNIQUE

We perform a medial approach from the medial maleollus up to the ATT distal insertion. The PTT is explored. If there is substantial damage, it is resected; otherwise, its borders are fixed to other flexors, remembering that they are synergic. The ATT is then freed beginning in its distal insertion until the ankle, moving it without detaching it (**Figs. 1–3**).

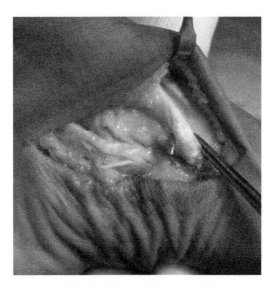

Fig. 1. The ATT.

A horizontal cut is performed over the inner side of the navicular, at a central point between the dorsal and the sole of the foot, following its horizontal axis. Two osteoperiosteal flaps are carved—upper (**Fig. 4**) and lower (**Fig. 5**)—using a chisel and trying to carve them deep, so that the navicular remains with the entire cancellous

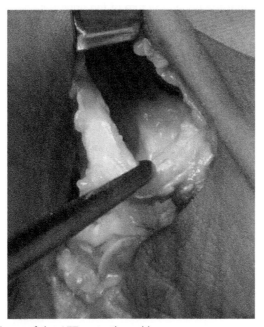

Fig. 2. Proximal release of the ATT up to the ankle.

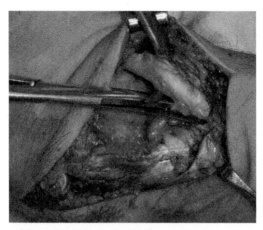

Fig. 3. Distal release of the ATT, without detaching it.

bone exposed. A slot is sculpted along the navicular, as plantar as possible (**Fig. 6**). The proximal side of the navicular slot is made round to avoid a possible lesion caused by the sharp edge to the ATT while being translocated to its new position.

The ATT is lowered and located in the slot sculpted in the navicular in the inner edge of the foot (**Fig. 7**) and both osteoperiosteal flaps are closed, tensing them and suturing them over the tendon (**Fig. 8**). The ATT is pulled underneath the navicular, because it is a tremendous support for the medial arch of the foot.

Depending on the surgeon's preference, it is possible to add in the depth of the canal an anchor, with 1 or 2 metal spears, if there are doubts that the osteoperiosteal flap of fragile structure may not be able to keep the tendon in its new position. It is worth remembering that the bone structure of the adult patients is not the same as that of younger patients, for whom the procedure was originally described.

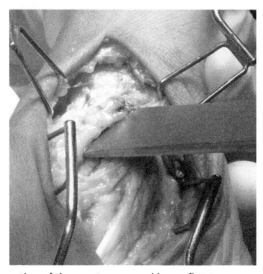

Fig. 4. Carving or creation of the great upper and lower flaps.

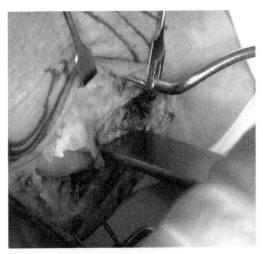

Fig. 5. The lower flap leans the entire medial capsular–ligamentous apparatus.

The patient is kept in postoperative care immobilized with an open cast. After 15 days, the splint and the skin stitches are removed, and the patient is immobilized again, this time with a closed cast with the ankle in neutral position. One month after the operation, the patient is allowed to bear weight completely. Two months after surgery, the cast is removed and an Arizona splint is applied for another month, and the patient begins hydrotherapy to start mobilizing the foot.

It was necessary to modify Young's original procedure. Young's procedure[2] sculpts a vertical slot in the navicular, so that the ATT has a horizontal trajectory under the navicular

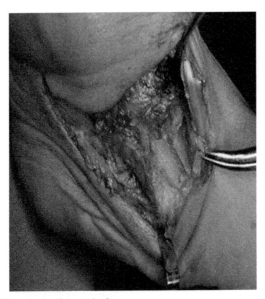

Fig. 6. Creation of the slot in the navicular.

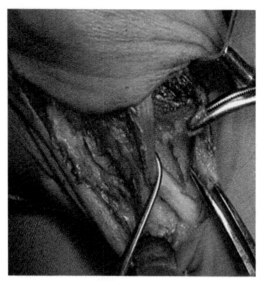

Fig. 7. The ATT is lowered, changing its route.

and vertical in its proximal sector. However, we found it difficult to lower the ATT given that, even when this foot is mobile, it does not present the flexibility of a child. Therefore, it was necessary to make a horizontal trajectory, keeping it as plantar as possible so that it supports the internal and plantar capsular and ligamentous apparatus.

The second reason why the trajectory was altered was that the majority of these patients having a very osteoporotic navicular, which may break while trying to sculpt the vertical slot. Is this isolated procedure enough to correct all the components of the

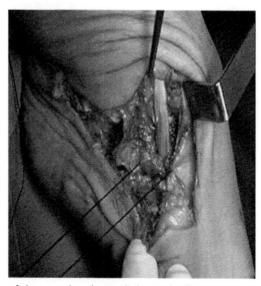

Fig. 8. Overlapping of slots, tensing the medial capsular ligamentous apparatus.

pathology? The purpose of this tendinous translocation is to find a substitute for the insufficient PTT and achieve an adequate muscle balance.

1. We must take into account that the ATT is not detached, so its function mechanism is still active. Only its distal 10 or 15 cm where moved to redirect it, so that the proximal area has a more vertical trajectory in the inner edge of the foot. Because of this trajectory change, its lifting action increases the upward pull of the inner arch, reinforcing the action that the tibialis posterior had in its sling function at the level of the navicular.[18]
2. The horizontal trajectory of the ATT is performed with an almost plantar route, and it is covered by osteoperiosteal flaps that are tensed on top of it, constituting a powerful inner capsular–tendinous–ligamentous support.
3. The ATT translocation makes this tendon unable to lift the first metatarsal, causing it to pull the navicular. Therefore, an insufficiency of the ATT is created, which results in a predominance of the peroneus lateral longus that descends and prones the forefoot causing an active increase in the height of the arch in the inner side of the foot.

What are the advantages over other procedures? First, The muscle used is not detached; therefore, it works actively. Second, it achieves a good muscle balance, which results in an improvement of the medial arch providing it with active components, reinforcing the action of the PTT and granting an insufficiency of the ATT, which results in a predominance of the peroneus lateral longus. Third, it reinforces soft parts of the plantar and medial sector. Fourth, it does not sacrifice the joint mobility. Finally, it is an efficient procedure that acts anatomically and functionally.

COMPARISON WITH OTHER PROCEDURES
Flexor Digitorum Longus

Although the flexor digitorum longus (FDL) is a plantar flexor and supinator, moving it to the navicular results in a reinforcement of the insufficient PTT, but diminishes the flexor–plantar action, which is very important.[19–23] It is worth remembering that the FDL is one third of the size of the PTT and capable of applying one third of the force of the PTT; therefore the question posed is this: Is this tendon enough to transpose or perform a tenodesis?

Comparative Force and Tendon Excursion

Silver and associates[24] affirm the values in **Table 1**. The ATT provides for 80% of the dorsiflexion force of the ankle. Hintermann and co-workers[25] conducted an in vitro

| Table 1 | | |
| Comparative force and tendon excursion | | |
	Force	Excursion
Tibialis anterior tendon	5.6	2.9
Posterior tibial tendon	6.4	1.6
Flexor hallucis longus	3.6	1.7
Flexor digitorum longus	1.8	1.2
Peroneus longus	5.5	1.6
Peroneus brevis	2.6	1.4
Achilles	49.1	4.0

study of foot movement and tendon excursion. They speculated that rotation is provided by a low insertion and high excursion, whereas the stabilizing function is more effective with several insertions acting to move bones together. The stabilizing function was attributed mainly to those muscles with numerous insertions and low maximum tendon excursion (eg, the PTT). The major contribution of the PTT to foot stability results from the locking-in mechanism of the midfoot.

The main function of the flexor hallucis longus and FDL may be attributed to toe flexion–extension. They additionally exert an inverting effect on the rearfoot. They do not have such influence on midfoot motion; their stabilizing function over of the foot eversion–inversion axis may be substantially less than the one of the tibialis posterior. In relation to the tibialis anterior inversion–eversion axes, it is not as high as the one the tibialis posterior can produce.

The ATT has an invertor moment about 0.6 when the referential is tibialis posterior (as the FLD). Its moment arm is twice as long with regards to the flexion–extension axis, making it a strong extensor. In an attempt to increase the leverage as an invertor, ATT transfer may, therefore, not be an adequate method for the treatment of FFD. Such surgery may result additionally in the loss of the extensor function.

Our hypothesis is that with the translocation, the force of the ATT will be canalized as an invertor and the loss of its extensor force will help to correct the forefoot supination. Cobb[26] described a method of reconstruction in Johnson and Strom type II PTT[27] dysfunction, performing a transfer of a split of the ATT.[28,29] In 1990, Helal[30] described satisfactory results in 5 of 8 patients with use of the split ATT procedure in patients with a stage 2 PTT.

The goal of the Cobb procedure[26] is to reconstruct a functional ATT associated with a torn PTT. In the Cobb method, half of the ATT is left attached at its insertion and it is passed throughout a hole drilled in the cuneiform to the PTT compartment, performing an anastomosis in the proximal end of the PTT. The advantage of the Cobb procedure over the FDL is that the loss of a plantar flexor is avoided, what at the same time, generates a partial insufficiency of the ATT when dividing it in half. Later, this produces the fall of the first metatarsal and the pronation of the forefoot.

Mann and Thompson[22] affirm that performing the slot in the cuneiform instead of the navicular increases the lever arm of the transferred tendon and prevents any collapse in the navicular–cuneiform, which is sometimes associated with the collapse of the talonavicular joint.

Baravarian and co-workers[31] said that the Cobb technique is not ideal for all patients because if the muscle–tendinous unit of the tibialis posterior is left nonfunctional or severely scarred owing to prolonged disuse, the anastomosis will not have a proper functioning because it depends on the condition of the tibial posterior muscle (PTT) for its action. Valdebarrano and associates[32] carried out a study to determine the recovery potential of the PTT after tendon rupture. They state that the recovery potential of the PTT seemed to be significant even after delayed repair.

Knupp and Hinterman[33] carried out a prospective study with the Cobb procedure and included 22 consecutive patients with supple flatfoot deformity caused by PTT dysfunction. Average follow-up was 24 months. The overall clinical results obtained were excellent (41%), good (54%), fair (5%), and poor (none). They stated that the advantage is that the Cobb procedure decreases the tension of the ATT.

This dynamic correction may allow the patient to adapt the forefoot to the ground as required. The Cobb procedure may, to a certain extent, correct the "functional amputation" of the first ray that occurs with the forefoot supination deformity.[33] The resulting improved and preserved weight distribution in the forefoot is thought to give the patient better control and stability in stance of gait.

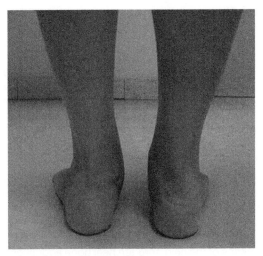

Fig. 9. Preoperative left FFD. Too many toes sign.

BONE PROCEDURES THAT MAY BE ASSOCIATED WITH YOUNG'S TECHNIQUE
Calcaneal Osteotomy

Osteotomies provide the foot with a more stable posture. It allows the transferred or translocated tendon to function more effectively.[34,35] The biomechanical improvement of

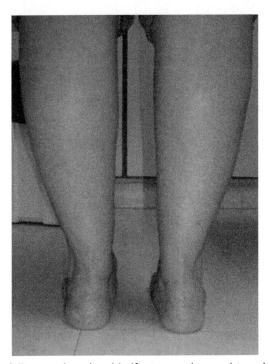

Fig. 10. At 7 years' follow up, the valgus hindfoot correction persists and the too many toes sign disappears.

a medial translocation of the calcaneus is believed to be a result of the restoration of the gastrosoleus medial axis with the ankle joint.[36] As a result of the change of the subtalar vector, the hindfoot forces change diminishing the stress in the internal repair, thereby protecting the tendinous transference.

This osteotomy is extra-articular, and for that reason it does not impact or compromise any joint, avoiding rigidity. As we said, a fully movable foot is fundamental for Young's procedure to be effective. Moreover, the internal displacement of the calcaneus bone reduces stress over the deltoid ligament. For all these reasons, we prefer this technique over other procedures.

Lengthening of the External Column

This technique is used to correct forefoot abduction, produced in FFD, determining a shortening of the external column.[37-40] The technique is carried out by lengthening the mentioned sector by distraction, placing a graft in the calcaneal osteotomy, or elongation at the level of the calcaneal–cuboid joint and placing a graft in it. Evans, modified[41] by Mosier,[42] states that the anterior calcaneal osteotomy permits the internal rotation by means of the heel, through heel bone adduction with simultaneous supination and plantar flexion. He also documented that it corrects the radiologic values of FDD, even the talonavicular coverage; however, the mechanism is unknown. What are the drawbacks of this technique? It is a purely morphologic correction; shortening of the external column is caused by a functional lengthening of the medial

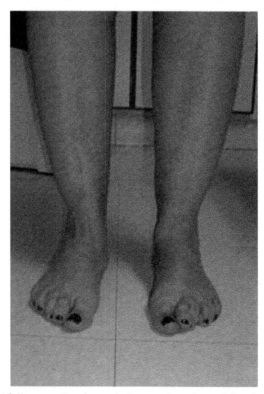

Fig. 11. At 7 years' follow-up. Good morphology and no signs of forefoot abduction.

column produced by the insufficiency of the PTT and the medial capsule ligament elements. Our hypothesis is that if we are able to control the medial functional insufficiency we will achieve the coverage of the head of the talus with the navicular, not anatomically but functionally.

Following authors such as Coetzee and Castro,[36] we agree that this technique causes improper rotation of the forefoot in varus and supination, and probably worsens the supination already present in the forefoot, which is what Young's procedure tries to correct. Lengthening the external column increases pressure over the joints, which may cause a rigidity not adequate when combining this technique with Young's, given that Young's procedure requires a mobile foot to obtain successful results. Mosier and colleagues[42] state that 65% of patients present with calcaneocuboid arthritis, loss of correction over time, and loss of mobility in the rest of the joints of the hind foot owing to such arthritis.

The placement of the graft in the external sector,[36] near the posterior subtalar joint, produces an impact over this joint, generating sinus tarsi pain. Nonunion is still the most common complication. It occurs in 10% to 20% of cases and usually requires a revision procedure.[36]

Cuneiform Osteotomy With Bone Graft

Supination of the forefoot in this pathology is a complication that has not been considered by many authors. However, many others propose acting over the first cuneiform to correct it, by means of a cuneiform osteotomy with bone graft. This technique[43] performs an osteotomy in the center of the first cuneiform, placing a triangular graft in the dorsal base, trying to provide flexion to the unstable medial

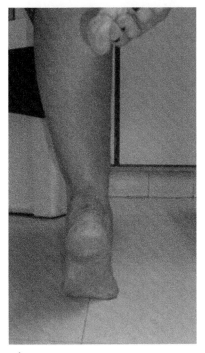

Fig. 12. Absence of tip toe sign.

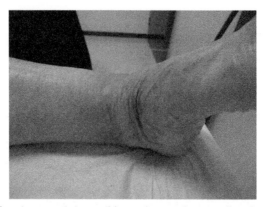

Fig. 13. With the foot in varus, it is possible to observe the new direction of the ATT.

column of the foot and correct supination. However, we insist that it is purely an anatomic correction, because it does not add motors to contribute with plantar flexion, as Young's procedure does, generating an insufficiency of the anterior tibialis tendon.

Talonavicular Arthrodesis

Young's procedure is contraindicated in a foot with some sort of rigidity.[44]

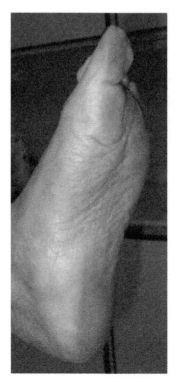

Fig. 14. Forefoot pronation.

Arthroerisis

The biomechanics of the implant function have not been fully elucidated. They present the problem that they may determine, eventually, a decrease in the subtalar mobility.[45,46] Schon[47] says that the arthroerisis seems beneficial with a low-risk profile. The high implant removal rate is a concern, but implant removal brings about a resolution of the pain without loss of correction.

In the future, better studies will help to define the outcomes, and determine whether it does not diminish the subtalar mobility or causes its arthritis.

MATERIAL AND METHODS

We retrospectively studies 35 patients with supple flatfoot deformity caused by PTT dysfunction treated with Young's procedure.[2] The operations were carried out between 1994 and 2010 with a minimum follow-up of 1 year, a maximum follow-up of 17 years, and median of 6.5 years.

There were 2 groups with similar characteristics in relation to gender, age, weight; and previous treatment (Young's procedure, 14 patients [42.4%] among others). Young's procedure and medial displacement calcaneal osteotomy 21 patients (57.6%). The American Orthopaedic Foot and Ankle Society score system[48] was used in the analysis of the results. This score increased from a preoperative value of 50.77% to 94.14% points at the latest follow-up. The postoperative score for Young's technique was 92.76 and Young's technique and calcaneal osteotomy was 95 points (**Figs. 9–16**).

The overall clinical results were graded as excellent (American Orthopaedic Foot and Ankle Society score, 100%) in 11 (31.43%). In this group, all patients were treated with Young's technique and calcaneal osteotomy. Results were good (score range, 90–99) in 17 (48.57%), fair (score range, 80–89) in 6 (17.14%), and

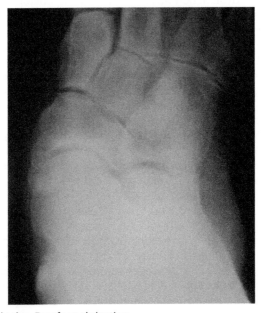

Fig. 15. Uncovered talus. Forefoot abduction.

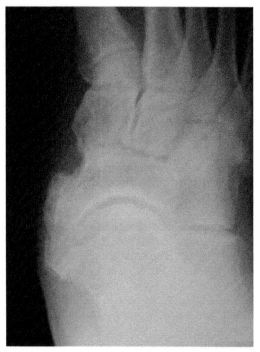

Fig. 16. Covered talus, 7 years postoperative.

poor (score, <80) in 1 (2.86%). The poor outcome was the only patient with PTT rupture. Clinical ATT dysfunction occurred in the early postoperative period. The patients had decreased tibial anterior tendon power, but after 6 months none had clinical ATT dysfunction.

No patient had first ray metatarsalgia caused by an ATT dysfunction at latest follow-up. Forefoot postoperative supination occurred in 6 patients (17.1%). In these cases, Young's technique was performed without medial displacement calcaneal osteotomy. Although some patients had persistent forefoot supination and hindfoot valgus, 97% were satisfied with the results. They manifested they could feel the ground and, after surgery, recover foot control.

Of our cases, 85% had no pain and only 15% occasional and moderate pain. All patients were able to perform daily living activities without the use of canes and only 12% had some limitations at recreational activities. Postoperatively, 33 patients (94.2%) were able to wear shoes without insoles; 6 (17.1%) preferred to have insoles.

Comparing both groups, Young's procedure is useful to reconstruct a supple FFD, but additional procedures, such as medial displacement calcaneal osteotomy, should be considered to correct the entire deformity. Of our patients, 97% did not experience a progression of the flatfoot deformity at follow-up. This procedure improves functionality, gait capability, and subjective stability, which may be explained by an improved control of proprioception. In all, 97.1% of patients are satisfied with their results. We believe that Young's technique respects the anatomy and biomechanics of the foot to reach the necessary muscular balance.

SUMMARY

Young's procedure contains an action mechanism that works better than other techniques on the pathophysiology of FFD. It respects the anatomy and biomechanics of the foot to reach the necessary muscular balance. The benefits of this technique include that the ATT is not detached, so its function mechanism is still active; the new trajectory of the ATT provides a powerful sling function at the level of the navicular; and the horizontal trajectory of the ATT and the osteoperiosteal flaps constitute a powerful inner capsular–tendinous–ligamentous support. What is more, an insufficiency of the ATT is created, which results in a predominance of the peroneus lateral longus, that descends and prones the forefoot. Additional procedures, such as medial displacement calcaneal osteotomy, should be considered to correct the entire deformity. The combination of these techniques do not sacrifice the joint mobility.

ACKNOWLEDGMENTS

The authors thank María Noel Maquieira for translation of the manuscript.

REFERENCES

1. Ruiz S, Mauro L. Tratamiento quirúrgico del pie plano. Revista de Cirugía del Uruguay 1974;43:543–5.
2. Young CS. Operative treatment of pes planus. Surg Gynecol Obstet 1939;68:1099–101.
3. Van Boerum D, Sangeorzan B. Biomechanics and pathophysiology of flatfoot. Foot Ankle Clin 2003;8:419–30.
4. Navarro A. Nuevos conceptos sobre la fisiologia del pie. Deducciones patológicas Anales del Instituto de Clínica quirúrgica y cirugía experimental. Tomo 5. Montevideo: Rosgal; 1943. p. 9–81.
5. Mauro L. Biomecánica del pie plano estático en niños y adolescentes. In X Congreso Latinoamericano de Ortopedia y Traumatología. Río de Janeiro; 1977.
6. Kapandji JA. Miembro inferior. In: Cuadernos de fisiología articular, vol. 2. Barcelona: Toray-Masson; 1982. p. 136–219.
7. Llorens Isidro A, Nuñez Samper M, Llanos Alcazar LF, editors. Filogenia del pie. In: Biomecánica Medicina y Cirugía del pie. Barcelona: Masson; 1997. p. 8–13.
8. Ness ME, Long J, Marks R, et al. Foot and ankle kinematics in subjects with PTT dysfunction. Gait Posture 2008;27:331–9.
9. Cracchiolo A. Evaluation of spring ligament pathology in patients with posterior tibial tendon rupture, tendon transfer and ligament repair. Foot Ankle Clin 1997;2:297–309.
10. Giza E, Cush G, Schon L. The flexible flat foot in the adult. Foot Ankle Clin 2007;12:251–72.
11. Huang CK, Kitaoka HB, An KN. Biomechanics evaluation of longitudinal arch stability. Foot Ankle Int 1993;14:353–7.
12. Kitaoka HB, Ahn TK, Luo ZP, et al. Stability of the arch of the foot. Foot Ankle Int; 1997;18:644–8.
13. Otis JC. Clinical and applied biomechanics. In: Myerson M, editor. Foot and ankle disorders. Philadelphia: WB Saunders Company; 2000. p. 181–94.
14. DiGiovanni C, Langer P. The role of the isolated gastrocnemius and combined Achilles contractures in the flat foot. Foot Ankle Clin 2007;12:363–79.
15. Neptune RR, Kantz SA, Zajac FE. Contributions of the individual ankle plantar flexors to support forward progression and swing initiation during walking. J Biomech 2001;34:1387–98.

16. Bluman EM, Title CI, Myerson MS. Posterior tibial tendon rupture. A refined classification system. Foot Ankle Clin 2007;12:233–49.
17. Hintermann B, Gachter A. The first metatarsal rise sign. A simple sensitive sign of tibial posterior tendon dysfunction. Foot Ankle Int 1996;17:236–41.
18. El-Tayeby HM. The severe flexible flatfoot: a combined reconstructive procedure with rerouting of the tibialis anterior tendon. J Foot Ankle Surg 1999;38:41–9.
19. DiPaola M, Raikin S. Tendon transfers and realignment osteotomies for treatment of Stage II posterior tibial tendon dysfunction. Foot Ankle Clin 2007;12:273–82.
20. Guyton G, Jeng C, Krieger L, et al. Flexor digitorum longus transfer and medial displacement calcaneal osteotomy for posterior tibial tendon dysfunction. A middle-term clinical follow up. Foot Ankle Int 2001;22:627–63.
21. Thompson MR. Rupture of the posterior tibial tendon causing flat foot. Surgical treatment. J Bone Joint Surg Am 1985;67:556–61.
22. Myerson MS, Badekas A, Schon LC. Treatment of stage II posterior tibial tendon deficiency with flexor digitorum longus transfer and calcaneal osteotomy. Foot Ankle Int 2004;25:445–50.
23. Parsons S, Naim S, Richards P, et al. Correction and prevention of deformity in type II tibialis posterior dysfunction. Clin Orthop Relat Res 2010;468:1025–32.
24. Silver RL, de la Garza J, Rang M. The myth of muscle balance. A study of relative strengths and excursions of normal muscles about the foot and ankle. J Bone Joint Br 1985;67:432–7.
25. Hintermann B, Nigg BM, Sommer C. Foot movement and tendon excursion: an in vitro study. Foot Ankle Int 1994;15:386–95.
26. Cobb N. Tibialis posterior disorders. In: Helal B, Rowley DI, Cracchiolo A III, et al, editors. Surgery of disorders of the foot and ankle. London (UK): Martin Dunley; 1996. p. 291–301.
27. Johnson KA, Strom DE. Tibialis posterior tendon dysfunction. Clin Orthop Rel Res 1989;239:196–206.
28. Basmajian JV, Stecko G. The role of muscles in arch support of the foot J Bone Joint Surg 1963;45:1184–90.
29. Biga N, Moulier D, Mabit C. Pied plat valgus statique. EMQ. Paris: Elsevier; 1999.
30. Helal B. Cobb repair for tibialis posterior tendon rupture. J Foot Surg 1990;29:349–58.
31. Baravarian B, Zgonis T, Lowery C. Use of the Cobb procedure in the treatment of posterior tibial tendon dysfunction. Clin Podiatr Med Surg 2002:19:371–89.
32. Valdebarrano V, Hintermann B, Wischer T, et al. Recovery of the posterior tibial muscle after late reconstruction following tendon rupture. Foot Ankle Int 2004;25:85–95.
33. Knupp M, Hintermann B. The Cobb procedure for treatment of acquired flatfoot deformity associated with stage II insufficiency of the posterior tibial tendon. Foot Ankle Int 2007;28:416–21.
34. Hiller L, Pinney SJ. Surgical treatment of acquired flatfoot deformity: what is the state of practice among academic foot and ankle surgeons in 2002? Foot Ankle Int 2003;24:701–5.
35. Vora AM, Tien TR, Parks BG, et al. Correction of moderate and severe acquired flexible flatfoot with medializing calcaneal osteotomy and flexor digitorum longus transfer. J Bone Joint Surg Am 2006;88:1726–34.
36. Coetzee C, Castro M. The indications and biomechanical rationale for various hindfoot procedures in the treatment of posterior tibialis tendon dysfunction. Foot Ankle Clin 2003;8:453–9.
37. Anderson RB, Davis WH. Calcaneocuboid distraction arthrodesis for the treatment of the adult acquired flatfoot. The modified Evans procedure. Foot Ankle Clin 1996;1: 279–94.

38. Krans A, Louwerens JW, Anderson P. Adult acquired flexible flatfoot, treated by calcaneo-cuboid distraction arthrodesis, posterior tibial tendon augmentation, and percutaneous Achilles tendon lengthening: a prospective outcome study of 20 patients. Acta Orthop 2006;77:156–63.
39. Sands A, Tansey JP. Lateral column lengthening. Foot Ankle Clin 2007;12:301–30.
40. Sangeorzan B, Mosca V, Hansen ST. Effect of calcaneal lengthening on relationships among the hindfoot, midfoot, and forefoot. Foot Ankle Int 1993;14:136–41.
41. Evans D. Calcaneus valgus deformity. J Bone Joint Surg Br 1975;57:270–8.
42. Mosier SM, Pomeroy G, Manoli A. Pathoanatomy and etiology of posterior tibial tendon dysfunction. Clin Orthop Rel Res 1999;365:12–22.
43. Tankson CJ. The Cotton osteotomy: indications and techniques lengthening. Foot Ankle Clin 2007;12:309–16.
44. Cohen B, Ogden F. Medial column procedures in the acquired flatfoot deformity. Foot Ankle Clin 2007;12:287–301.
45. Giannini S, Ceccarelli F, Benedetti M. Surgical treatment of flexible flatfoot in children: a four years follow up study. J Bone Joint Surg Am 2001;83(Suppl 2):73–9.
46. Viladot A. Surgical treatment of the child flatfoot. Clin Orthop1992;283:34.
47. Schon L. Subtalar arthroerisis: a new exploration of an old concept. Foot Ankle Clin 2007;12:329–39.
48. Kitaoka HB, Alexander IJ, Adalaar RS, et al. Clinical rating systems for the ankle-hindfoot, midfoot, hallux and lesser toes. Foot Ankle Int 1994;15:349–53.

Calcaneal Osteotomy in the Treatment of Adult Acquired Flatfoot Deformity

Abhijit R. Guha, MBBS(Hons), MS(Orth), FRCS(Ed), FRCS(Tr & Orth)*,
Anthony M. Perera, MBChB, MRCS, MFSEM, PGDip (Med Law), FRCS (Orth)

KEYWORDS
- Adult acquired flatfoot • Arthrodesis • Lateral column lengthening
- Medial displacement calcaneal osteotomy • Tibialis posterior

KEY POINTS
- Adult acquired flatfoot deformity is a common problem after middle age.
- Failure of the tibialis posterior tendon, followed by the plantar calcaneonavicular ligament and the anterior fibers of the deltoid ligament, leads to deformity.
- Medial displacement calcaneal osteotomy (MDCO) is used in stage 2 deformity to correct the ground reaction force and prevents the heel from going into valgus. It converts the gastrosoleus from an evertor to an invertor of the heel.
- Lateral column lengthening procedures are used to correct forefoot abduction and uncovering of the talar head.
- Medial displacement calcaneal osteotomy may be used in combination with lateral column lengthening to improve correction.

Adult acquired flatfoot deformity (AAFD) is a chronic, debilitating condition common beyond middle age. It is characterized by a painful flattening of the medial longitudinal arch and has been referred to as posterior tibial tendon deficiency. However, in recognition of the fact that other structures such as the plantar calcaneonavicular (spring) ligament and the deltoid ligament were also involved, the nomenclature has been changed to AAFD.

Weakness of the tibialis posterior leads to the inability to invert the heel taking it from valgus in the midstance phase of gait into inversion. This is key to initiating heel rise by changing the line of pull of the Achilles; it also locks the midfoot, providing a rigid lever for push-off. Without this, the transverse tarsal joint axes remain in alignment and there is no longer a rigid lever arm for the gastrocnemius muscle to

Department of Trauma and Orthopaedics, University Hospital of Wales, Heath Park, Cardiff, Wales, CF14 4XW, UK
* Corresponding author.
E-mail address: footandanklesurgery@gmail.com

Foot Ankle Clin N Am 17 (2012) 247–258
doi:10.1016/j.fcl.2012.02.003
1083-7515/12/$ – see front matter Crown Copyright © 2012 Published by Elsevier Inc. All rights reserved.

contract against in the heel rise phase of gait. This subsequently puts a repetitive load on the medial supporting structures, leading to the eventual degeneration and weakening of the tibialis posterior, spring ligament and the anterior fibers of the deltoid ligament.

Failure of these structures leads to the classic pes planovalgus deformity. The consequent shortening of the gastrocnemius further exacerbates the flattening of the medial longitudinal arch. In the presence of a short gastrocnemius muscle, terminal dorsiflexion of the ankle is achieved by rotation around the talonavicular joint; over time, this joint becomes subluxed. This peritalar instability results in the navicular moving superiorly, laterally, and supinating further, contributing to instability of the medial column and the collapse of the arch.

CLASSIFICATION

The condition was originally classified by Johnson and Strom[1] into 3 stages with a fourth stage added later.[2] The use of a calcaneal osteotomy is most pertinent to stage 2, although there are rare instances in stages 3 and 4 when this may be required in addition to fusion surgery to achieve full correction. For instance, when there is a severe deformity but insufficient bone stock to perform the correction purely through a fusion.

Stage 2 disease represents tendon failure in a planovalgus foot that has not yet become rigid or degenerate and with normal ankle alignment. The aim of surgery is functional reconstruction and rebalancing of the foot with a tendon transfer. There is clear evidence that a bony heel correction is a key part of the operative management of stage 2 disease. However, the issue with this classification system is that stage 2 includes a significant variation in the type and severity of deformity of the midfoot and hindfoot. Therefore, this stage has been further subdivided by various authors, depending on the degree of coverage of the talonavicular joint and forefoot varus (Anderson, Instructional Course Lectures, 2003), or the degree of resting supination of the forefoot and its correctability in the Truro classification.[3] Myerson and colleagues[4] have proposed a detailed classification of AAFD that would help to guide the surgeon to decide on the appropriate surgical options available at the various stages of the disease. This is a comprehensive classification, incorporating the wide variety of presentations in each stage and helps to individualize treatment according to the patient's particular pathology. This morphologic approach aids with preoperative planning in selecting the most appropriate type of bony correction: Medial Displacement Calcaneal Osteotomy (MDCO), lateral column lengthening, a combination, or arthroereisis (not strictly an osteotomy but included here for completeness; **Table 1**).

OPERATIVE MANAGEMENT

Failure of nonoperative management is the commonest indication to proceed to operative management. Most patients with AAFD requiring operative intervention have stage 2 deformity. The operative management of stage 2 deformity has undergone a change in direction over the last 30 years.[5] Joint-preserving procedures, which aim to realign the hindfoot and augment the dysfunctional tibialis posterior tendon, have now taken precedence over hindfoot fusion procedures, which are now used if the hindfoot joints are already arthritic or in the revision/salvage setting. Before proceeding to surgery, one must consider the flexibility of the foot, the apex of the deformity, the condition of the tibialis posterior tendon, the spring ligament, the deltoid ligament, and presence of arthritis in the hindfoot joints. Augmentation of the dysfunctional tibialis posterior tendon by transfer of the flexor digitorum longus

Table 1 Comprehensive staging with pathology and treatment options in AFFD			
Stage	Subdivision	Pathology	Recommendation
2	A	Flexible hindfoot valgus with	
		Flexible forefoot varus	Medial posting/brace + tendoachilles lengthening if forefoot varus corrects only in equinus
		Fixed forefoot varus	MDCO (arthroereisis) + FDL transfer + Cotton osteotomy if fixed forefoot varus
	B	Forefoot abduction (at transverse tarsal, first TMT joint or both)	
		Talar head uncovering <40%	MDCO + FDL transfer
		Talar head uncovering >40%	FDL transfer + Lateral column lengthening ± MDCO/arthroereisis (if residual heel valgus)
	C	Medial ray instability	
		Persistent forefoot varus after correction of heel	
		Talonavicular/naviculocuneiform/ first TMT joint level	Fusion of appropriate joint if arthritic/Cotton osteotomy

Abbreviations: Cotton osteotomy, opening wedge medial cuneiform osteotomy; FDL, flexor digitorum longus; TMT, tarsometatarsal.

Adapted from Bluman EM, Title CI, Myerson MS. Posterior tibial tendon rupture: a refined classification system. Foot Ankle Clin 2007;12:233–49.

(FDL) tendon does not seem to work when performed alone. This has been established by various authors in both clinical and laboratory studies.[6-8] Hence, corrective surgery most often involves a calcaneal osteotomy, repair of the spring ligament and talonavicular joint capsule (principal static restraints) and augmentation of the tibialis posterior with the FDL, flexor hallucis longus, or sometimes even the peroneus brevis. If the gastrocnemius muscle is contracted, a recession is performed to improve dorsiflexion at the ankle and reduce strain on the medial structures. Subtalar arthroereisis has also been advocated in the recent literature, to improve foot alignment by blocking rotation of the anterolateral talar body into the sinus tarsi and restricting subtalar joint movement preventing the peritalar instability.[9] The addition of the MDCO was the major step forward in the success of this surgery. Since then, other calcaneal osteotomies have been described.

MDCO
History

Gleich first attempted a calcaneal osteotomy to treat pes planus in 1893.[10] He attempted to restore a normal calcaneal pitch angle by performing a medial closing wedge osteotomy of the calcaneus and displacing the posterior fragment anteriorly, medially, and downward. Dwyer in 1960 proposed a lateral opening wedge osteotomy using tibial bone graft.

Biomechanics

MDCO allows greater correction of the deformity; most important, it changes the calcaneal axis protecting the soft tissue reconstruction using the ground reaction

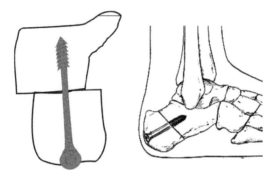

Fig. 1. Medial displacement calcaneal osteotomy.

force to prevent the heel from going into valgus. It also exerts a positive influence on walking dynamics. The MDCO (**Figs. 1** and **2**) restores the line of pull of the tendoachilles to the medial side of the subtalar joint axis and this helps to correct the valgus deformity of the hindfoot. The moment arm of the gastrosoleus in improved

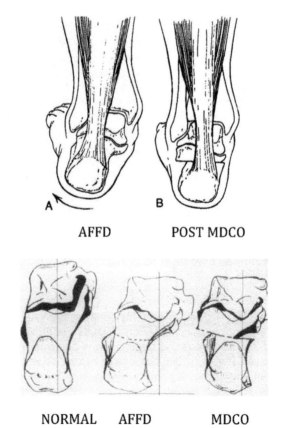

AFFD   POST MDCO

NORMAL   AFFD   MDCO

Fig. 2. Change in hindfoot axis after medial displacement calcaneal osteotomy.

and it is converted from an evertor in the deformed foot to an invertor of the heel in the corrected one.

MDCO has been reported to reduce the contact stresses at the tibiotalar joint and it is hoped that this would protect the ankle joint from degeneration in the future.[11] Other cadaveric studies have reported an increase in the peak pressure over the lateral forefoot and heel after MDCO.[12] Translation of 10 mm substantially decreases the load on the first metatarsal, medial arch, and the moment at the talonavicular joint, and increases the load on the lateral foot,[12] reversing the change in distribution of force that occurs in a failed tibialis posterior tendon.

Indications and Outcomes

Koutsogiannis[13] reintroduced the MDCO for treatment of AAFD in 1971. Since then, many authors including Myerson and colleagues,[4] Pomeroy and Manoli,[14] Fayazi and associates,[15] Wacker and co-workers,[16] Guyton and colleagues,[17] and Sammarco and Hockenbury[18] have published good results after MDCO, tendon transfer (either FDL or flexor hallucis longus), and spring ligament repair for the treatment of AAFD. MDCO is now recognized as an established procedure for surgical treatment of AAFD.

MDCO can be used in any situation where hindfoot valgus is present and protection of the medial soft tissues is required. Classically, it is used in the surgical treatment of stage 2 disease, in combination with other procedures. A cadaveric study showed that MDCO with FDL transfer was adequate in moderate degrees of deformity, but in cases of severe deformity, additional procedures were required.[19] It can be used in combination with tenosynovectomy of the tibialis posterior tendon in stage 1 disease and also with triple fusion, spring ligament reconstruction, and deltoid ligament reconstruction.

MDCO is a straightforward, reproducible, reliable procedure with predictable results. Myerson presented 120 patients treated in this way with marked improvement in pain and function in 90%.[4] However, radiologic arch improvement is not always achieved with this protocol; other series have shown that, despite good clinical outcomes, radiologic improvement in the arch itself may not be achieved in 0% to 75%. It has been noted that even this improvement in the radiologic parameters can be lost with the passage of time.[20] Furthermore, although there may be improvement in the radiographic height and alignment of the medial longitudinal arch in some patients, the outer appearance is significantly changed in only 4% of patients.[17]

Technique

The calcaneus is exposed through an oblique incision in line with the osteotomy or an extended lateral approach (**Fig. 3**A) with development of a full thickness flap anteriorly. The oblique incision allows a direct approach to the lateral calcaneal wall and is made parallel to the posterior facet of the subtalar joint and 2 cm posterior to it. A subperiosteal elevation is performed and soft tissue retractors are placed in the soft areas at either end of the incision.

The extended lateral approach is a radical anatomic dissection of a flap involving the skin, fascia, and local muscle with its blood supply. It exploits the watershed between the cutaneous supply of the posterior peroneal artery superiorly and the lateral plantar artery inferiorly. In contrast with the direct lateral approach, damage to the sural nerve is reduced and wound healing is not a concern.[21-24] The location of the skin incision is critical if damage to the sural nerve is to be avoided. The proximal arm of the incision runs almost to the midline posteriorly, staying away from the sural nerve. Care must be taken while dissecting around the peroneal tubercle to protect the peroneal tendons and the sural nerve is again potentially in danger at the distal

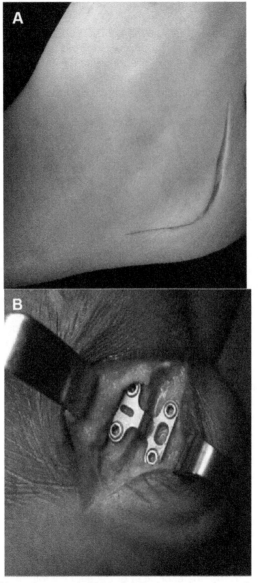

Fig. 3. (*A*) Extended lateral approach (*B*) Medial displacement calcaneal osteotomy held with step locking plate.

limb of the incision.[22] The extended lateral approach affords excellent exposure of the entire lateral wall of the calcaneus.[25]

The lateral wall of the tuberosity is exposed and Hohman retractors are placed on the dorsal and plantar aspects of the tuberosity. The dorsal retractor protects the Achilles tendon attachment, and the inferior one protects the plantar fascia. The osteotomy is started with an oscillating saw blade at a 90° angle to lateral wall if translation without plantarflexion is planned and at a right angle to the calcaneal axis (parallel to the posterior facet). A chevron-shaped osteotomy has been proposed as a more stable construct.

Completion of the medial cortex is done in a carefully controlled manner using a broad osteotome. The medial periosteum is then released on either side with an elevator. Displacement of at least 10 to 12 mm can be achieved after gentle sustained stretching of the medial soft tissues using a laminar spreader. The osteotomy can be fixed with either lag screws or step plates with locking screws (see **Fig. 3**B). It is important to hold the foot in dorsiflexion while fixing the osteotomy to compress the bony surfaces together.

Crushplasty of the prominent lateral edge has been recommended to avoid peroneal tendon pathology and sural nerve irritation. Lateral step plates are easy to apply, but can be prominent and preclude the use of a crushplasty. One to two 6.5-mm screws allow compression, easier soft tissue closure, and crushplasty, but can be prominent on the back of the heel.

The osteotomy is most often done in addition to other procedures that require immobilization of the limb in a plaster cast. However, after an isolated osteotomy, weight bearing may be allowed from 2 weeks; however, when a tendon transfer or spring ligament repair has also been undertaken, weight bearing is allowed after 4 to 6 weeks.

Complications

Nonunion is extremely rare and malunion can be avoided by good fixation and controlling the amount of bony contact that is maintained. A correction of 10 to 15 mm allows more than 50% contact and, thus, a stable construct.

Complications mainly involve the soft tissue structures on the medial side. Injury to the medial neurovascular bundle can be avoided by support under the distal tibia so that the medial ankle is unsupported, avoiding pressure on the medial structures. A pulsing action is used on the saw to cut to the far cortex and then broaching the medial cortex with an osteotome in a controlled fashion.

Sporadic case reports of injury to medial structures after calcaneal osteotomy appear in the literature. Tibial nerve palsy,[26] pseudoaneurysm of the posterior tibial artery and arteriovenous fistula,[27] and lateral plantar artery pseudoaneurysm[28] have been reported. A cadaveric study reported that a minimum of 2 medial structures crossed the osteotomy site at various positions. In most cases, branches of the lateral plantar nerve and the posterior tibial artery were involved.[29] The calcaneal sensory branch and the second branch of the lateral plantar nerve (Baxter's nerve) crossed the osteotomy site in 86% and 95% of specimens, respectively.[30] Injury to these branches may result in postoperative medial hindfoot pain. The authors recommended completion of the medial cortex of the osteotomy in a carefully controlled manner.

Limitations

MDCO does not correct forefoot abduction and uncovering of the talonavicular joint. To improve this, a lengthening procedure of the lateral column needs to be undertaken. This involves either a lengthening osteotomy through the anterior aspect of the calcaneus or a distraction arthrodesis of the calcaneocuboid joint if this joint has evidence of arthritic changes.

Another potential criticism is that it inconsistently restores the height of the medial longitudinal arch.[31] Wacker and co-workers[16] showed that, despite good early success, in 75% there was a recurrence there was a 10% recurrence rate at 3 to 5 years. It is not clear whether this is related to the degree of correction of the foot.

LATERAL COLUMN LENGHTENING OSTEOTOMY
History

Lateral column lengthening with tibialis posterior augmentation has also been used to correct stage 2 AAFD. The concept of lateral column was introduced by Evans.[32] He observed that, in patients with clubfeet, adduction of the forefoot could be corrected by shortening of the lateral column. Conversely, he proposed lengthening of the lateral column to correct forefoot abduction in congenital spastic flatfoot. He thus introduced the classic Evans osteotomy to lengthen the lateral column. This concept was later applied to correction of the adult flatfoot.[33] This aspect will be dealt with in detail in another article by Calder and colleagues elsewhere in this issue.

DOUBLE CALCANEAL OSTEOTOMY

This includes a MDCO along with a lateral column lengthening osteotomy of the calcaneus.

Biomechanics

These osteotomies evolved to correct 2 major aspects of AAFD. They incorporate a MDCO to correct hindfoot valgus with a lateral column lengthening to correct forefoot abduction and increase arch height. Moreover, the aim is to share the amount of correction between the 2 sites, reducing the pressures in each area. This can result in a more anatomic correction of the deformity and may further decrease the load on the dysfunctional posteromedial structures.

Indications and Outcomes

When used in combination with FDL transfer, there is symptomatic pain relief and the correction obtained has been noted to be lasting at intermediate follow-up.[32,33] There is little published on this technique.

MALERBA OSTEOTOMY
History

Malerba and De Marchi[34] advocated the use of calcaneal osteotomies in both varus and valgus deformities of the hindfoot. They noted that preservation of the subtalar joint and correction of its biomechanics afforded a positive influence on walking dynamics. Malerba and De Marchi described a Z osteotomy of the retrothalamic portion of the calcaneus (**Fig. 4**). This combines a medial displacement of the calcaneal tuberosity and lateral column lengthening through an extensile approach.

Technique

The calcaneus is approached directly through an oblique incision parallel and distal to the peroneal tendons, thereby reducing risk of injury to the peroneal tendons or the

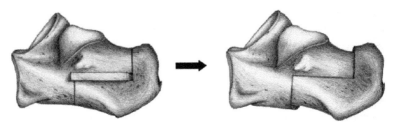

Fig. 4. Malerba Z osteotomy.

sural nerve. The osteotomy is performed using an oscillating saw and completed with an osteotome to protect the medial neurovascular structures. There are 3 osteotomic sections, similar in length and at right angles to each other. The central horizontal limb is at least 1.5 cm long, parallel to the weight bearing surface and distal to the peroneal tubercle, avoiding the need to expose the peroneal tendons. The proximal vertical limb exits into the dorsal concavity of the calcaneus between the attachment of the Achilles tendon and the posterior facet of the subtalar joint, whereas the distal vertical limb reaches the plantar cortex immediately anterior to the tuberosity, keeping well away from the calcaneocuboid joint.

This osteotomy allows the calcaneal tuberosity to be shifted medially or laterally; removal of a laterally based wedge adds to the correction of heel varus in pes cavus surgery. The osteotomy incorporates a large bony surface and its inherent stability encourages early consolidation. It is held with staples or screws and plaster immobilization is not necessary unless required by other associated procedures. Full weight bearing is usually possible within 6 weeks. Malerba osteotomy is a simple technique with limited risk of injury to the peroneal tendons or sural nerve and affords excellent potential to correct deformity on the frontal plane.

ARTHROEREISIS SCREW

Although this is not strictly a calcaneal osteotomy, it is included because it is used for a similar effect. It is perhaps the most controversial of the techniques described and is primarily indicated in the skeletally immature patient with dorsolateral peritalar instability. In this group, it is theorized that the implant blocks heel valgus and thus allows the foot to remodel with growth; nonetheless, it has been used in adults.

Biomechanics

In addition to correcting heel alignment, a 6-mm arthroereisis screw is successful at reversing the transfer in load to the medial foot that occurs with a tibialis posterior tendon dysfunction in a biomechanical model. The load on the first metatarsal, medial arch and talonavicular moment was reduced significantly.[35]

Indications and Outcomes

An arthroereisis screw can correct only mild deformity; therefore, it may have a role in the management of patients with little or no deformity and those in whom an adjunct to osteotomy is required. It may not correct the arch; the intention is really to block pronation protecting the medial tissues.

Complications

Despite the ease of insertion and ability to correct mild heel valgus complications are common. Needleman[36] reported that at 44 months 46% had sinus tarsi pain. Instability of the implant, pain, stiffness, and failure to improve deformity are also common.

SUMMARY

Calcaneal osteotomies are an essential part of our current armamentarium in the treatment of AAFD. Soft tissue correction or bony realignment alone have failed to adequately correct the deformity[37]; therefore, both procedures are used simultaneously to achieve long-term correction. Medial displacement and lateral column lengthening osteotomies in isolation or in combination and the Malerba osteotomy have been employed along with soft tissue balancing to good effect by various authors. The goal is to create a stable bony configuration with adequate soft tissue balance to maintain dynamic equilibrium in the hindfoot.

In "pronatory syndromes," the relation of the osteotomy to the posterior subtalar facet modifies the biomechanics of the hindfoot in different ways. Anterior calcaneal osteotomies correct deformities in the transverse plane (forefoot abduction), whereas posterior tuberosity osteotomies result in "varization" of the calcaneus and correct the frontal plane deformity.

The choice of osteotomy depends on the plane of the dominant deformity. If the subtalar axis is more horizontal than normal, transverse plane movement is cancelled out and the frontal plane eversion–inversion is predominant. The patient presents with marked hindfoot valgus without significant forefoot abduction. Conversely, if the subtalar axis is more vertical than normal, transverse plane movement is predominant and the patient presents with forefoot abduction and instability of the medial midtarsal joints, although without significant hindfoot valgus. In this situation, a lateral column lengthening procedure is recommended to decrease the uncovering of the talar head and improve the height of the arch while correcting the forefoot abduction. With a predominant frontal plane deformity, medialization of the calcaneal tuberosity is used to displace the calcaneal weight bearing axis medially, aligning it with the tibial axis and restoring the function of the gastrosoleus as a heel invertor. An essential prerequisite for this is the absence of arthritis affecting the subtalar joint. The Achilles tendon may need to be lengthened at the same time.

REFERENCES

1. Johnson KA, Strom DE. Tibialis posterior tendon dysfunction. Clin Orthop Relat Res 1989;239:196–206.
2. Bluman EM, Title CI, Myerson MS. Posterior tibial tendon rupture: a refined classification system. Foot Ankle Clin 2007;12:233–49.
3. Parsons S, Naim S, Richards PJ, et al. Correction and prevention of deformity in type II tibialis posterior dysfunction. Clin Orthop Relat Res 2010;468:1025–32.
4. Myerson MS, Badekas A, Schon LC. Treatment of stage II posterior tibial tendon deficiency with flexor digitorum longus tendon transfer and calcaneal osteotomy. Foot Ankle Int 2004;25:445–50.
5. Pinney SJ, Lin SS. Current concept review: acquired adult flatfoot deformity. Foot Ankle Int 2006;27:66–75.
6. Mann RA, Thompson FM. Rupture of the posterior tibial tendon causing flat foot. Surgical treatment. J Bone Joint Surg Am 1985;67:556–61.
7. Kitaoka HB, Luo ZP, An KN. Reconstruction operations for acquired flatfoot: biomechanical evaluation. Foot Ankle Int 1998;19:203–7.
8. Hill K, Saar WE, Lee TH, et al. Stage II flatfoot: what fails and why. Foot Ankle Clin 2003;8:91–104.
9. Needleman RL. Current topic review: subtalar arthroereisis for the correction of flexible flatfoot. Foot Ankle Int 2005;26:336–46.
10. Haddad SL, Myerson MS, Younger A, et al. Symposium: adult acquired flatfoot deformity. Foot Ankle Int 2011;32:95–111.
11. Hadfield M, Snyder J, Liacouras P, et al. The effects of a medializing calcaneal osteotomy with and without superior translation on Achilles tendon elongation and plantar foot pressures. Foot Ankle Int 2005;26:365–70.
12. Arangio GA, Salathe EP. A biomechanical analysis of posterior tibial tendon dysfunction, medical displacement calcaneal osteotomy and flexor digitorum longus transfer in adult acquired flatfoot. Clin Biomech 2009;24:385–90.

13. Koutsogiannis E. Treatment of mobile flat foot by displacement osteotomy of the calcaneus. J Bone Joint Surg Br 1971;53:96–100.
14. Pomeroy GC, Manoli A. A new operative approach for flatfoot secondary to posterior tibial tendon insufficiency: a preliminary report. Foot Ankle Int 1997;18:206–12.
15. Fayazi AH, Nguyen HV, Juliano PJ. Intermediate term follow-up of calcaneal osteotomy and flexor digitorum longus transfer for treatment of posterior tibial tendon dysfunction. Foot Ankle Int 2002;23:1107–11.
16. Wacker JT, Hennessy MS, Saxby TS. Calcaneal osteotomy and transfer of the tendon of flexor digitorum longus for stage-II dysfunction of tibialis posterior. Three- to five-year results. J Bone Joint Surg Br 2002;84:54–8.
17. Guyton GP, Jeng C, Krieger LE, et al. Flexor digitorum longus transfer and medial displacement calcaneal osteotomy for posterior tibial tendon dysfunction: a middle-term clinical follow-up. Foot Ankle Int 2001;22:627–32.
18. Sammarco GJ, Hockenbury RT. Treatment of stage II posterior tibial tendon dysfunction with flexor hallucis longus transfer and medial displacement calcaneal osteotomy. Foot Ankle Int 2001;22:305–12.
19. Vora AM, Tien TR, Parks BG, et al. Correction of moderate and severe acquired flexible flatfoot with medializing calcaneal osteotomy and flexor digitorum longus transfer. J Bone Joint Surg Am 2006;88:1726–34.
20. Bolt PM, Coy S, Toolan BC. A comparison of lateral column lengthening and medial translational osteotomy of the calcaneus for the reconstruction of adult acquired flatfoot. Foot Ankle Int 2007;28:1115–23.
21. Freeman BJ, Duff S, Allen PE, et al. The extended lateral approach to the hindfoot. Anatomical basis and surgical implications. J Bone Joint Surg Br 1998;80:139–42.
22. Eastwood DM, Irgau I, Atkins RM. The distal course of the sural nerve and its significance for incisions around the lateral hindfoot. Foot Ankle 1992;13:199–202.
23. Harvey EJ, Grujic L, Early JS, et al. Morbidity associated with ORIF of intra-articular calcaneus fractures using a lateral approach. Foot Ankle Int 2001;22:868–73.
24. Gould N. Lateral approach to the os calcis. Foot Ankle 1984;4:218–20.
25. Benirschke SK, Sangeorzan BJ. Extensive intraarticular fractures of the foot. Surgical management of calcaneal fractures. Clin Orthop Relat Res 1993;292:128–34.
26. Krause FG, Pohl MJ, Penner MJ, et al. Tibial nerve palsy associated with lateralizing calcaneal osteotomy: case reviews and technical tip. Foot Ankle Int 2009;30:258–61.
27. Doty JF, Alvarez RG, Asbury BS, et al. Arteriovenous fistula and pseudoaneurysm of the posterior tibial artery after calcaneal slide osteotomy: a case report. Foot Ankle Int 2010;31:329–32.
28. Ptaszek AJ, Aminian A, Schneider JR, et al. Lateral plantar artery pseudoaneurysm after calcaneal osteotomy: a case report. Foot Ankle Int 2006;27:141–3.
29. Vermeulen K, Neven E, Vandeputte G, et al. Relationship of the scarf valgus-inducing osteotomy of the calcaneus to the medial neurovascular structures. Foot Ankle Int 2011;32:S540–4.
30. Greene DL, Thompson MC, Gesink DS, et al. Anatomic study of the medial neurovascular structures in relation to calcaneal osteotomy. Foot Ankle Int 2001;22:569–71.
31. Pomeroy GC, Pike RH, Beals TC, et al. Acquired flatfoot in adults due to dysfunction of the posterior tibial tendon. J Bone Joint Surg Am 1999;81:1173–82.
32. Evans D. Calcaneo-valgus deformity. J Bone Joint Surg Br 1975;57:270–8.
33. Sangeorzan BJ, Mosca V, Hansen ST. Effect of calcaneal lengthening on relationships among the hindfoot, midfoot, and forefoot. Foot Ankle 1993;14:136–41.
34. Malerba F, De Marchi F. Calcaneal osteotomies. Foot Ankle Clin 2005;10:523–40.

35. Arangio GA, Reinert KL, Salathe EP. A biomechanical model of the effect of subtalar arthrodesis on the adult flexible flat foot. Clin Biomech 2004;19:847–52.

36. Needleman RL. A surgical approach for flexible flatfeet in adults including a subtalar arthrodesis with the MBA sinus tarsi implant. Foot Ankle Int 2006;27:9–18.

37. Trnka HJ, Easley ME, Myerson MS. The role of calcaneal osteotomies for correction of adult flatfoot. Clin Orthop Relat Res 1999;365:50–64.

Lateral Column Lengthening Osteotomies

Andrew J. Roche, FRCS (Tr & Orth)*,
James D.F. Calder, MD, FRCS (Tr & Orth), FFSEM(UK)

KEYWORDS

- Column • Foot • Lateral • Osteotomy

KEY POINTS

- The adult acquired flatfoot deformity requires intimate knowledge of not only the anatomy of the foot, but also of the biomechanical interactions between the joints.
- Lateral column lengthening can be performed in isolation or combined with other procedures to improve foot position and function.
- Both calcaneocuboid distraction arthrodesis and Evans-type procedures can be used successfully to lengthen the lateral column.

In the development of the adult acquired pes planovalgus foot deformity, the lateral column becomes relatively shortened in relation to the medial column. This gives the clinical appearance of an abduction deformity of the forefoot at Choparts joint and a hindfoot calcaneovalgus deformity. The Chopart joint is the transitional link between the hindfoot and the forefoot and it serves to compensate the forefoot for the hindfoot position. In the weight-bearing position, the internal rotation of the tibia imposes an eversion force on the subtalar joint. This subtalar position ensures the Choparts joints are essentially co-linear and are free to make compensatory adjustments on weight-bearing. During heel-rise and toe-off, lateral rotation of the tibia affects the subtalar joint to invert shifting the Achilles tendon medially initiated by the tibialis posterior muscle. This produces a rigid lever through Choparts joint and restricts motion at these joints because the joint axes are no longer parallel. Any loss of this effect at the subtalar joint results in loss of this rigid lever effect and the subtalar joint remains everted. The Chopart joint does not lock and gradually the effect of this is abduction of the forefoot on a calcaneovalgus deformity with lateral rotation of the navicular on the talus. On plain radiographs, this can be clearly seen with loss of talonavicular

The authors have nothing to disclose.
Department of Trauma and Orthopaedic Surgery, Chelsea and Westminster Hospital NHS Foundation Trust, 369 Fulham Road, London, SW10 9NH, UK
* Corresponding author. 7 Orchard End, Rowledge, Farnham, GU10 4EE, UK.
E-mail address: andyortho@gmail.com

coverage on the anteroposterior view and loss of medial cuneiform to fifth metatarsal height or a relatively proximal calcaneocuboid joint to the talonavicular joint on the lateral view.

WHAT IS LATERAL COLUMN LENGTHENING?

The lateral column of the foot comprises the anterior facet of the calcaneus, its articulation with the cuboid and the fourth and fifth tarsometatarsal joints. Lateral column lengthening procedures are typically used in patients with a pes planovalgus deformity. Procedures can be carried out at any level of the lateral column, but typically include a medializing calcaneal osteotomy, a distraction calcaneocuboid arthrodesis, or a lengthening osteotomy of the anterior process of the calcaneus. The goals of any or all of these procedures is to treat the patients symptoms by alleviating any discomfort and correct the clinical deformity, which improves foot kinematics during the gait cycle and reduces the likelihood of rapid progression of the disorder with degenerative changes in the hindfoot and midfoot.

CALCANEAL ANTERIOR PROCESS LENGTHENING PROCEDURES
Brief History

It is fascinating to think that the origins of this procedure emanated from a mistake made by a surgeon during surgical correction of a clubfoot. In 1961, Dilwyn Evans published a series of relapsed clubfeet corrections.[1] Part of the surgery was to perform a calcaneocuboid shortening excision arthrodesis. In 2 cases, however, he noticed an overcorrection owing to excessive bone excision, which produced a convex medial border and calcaneovalgus. After attempted corrections with calcaneal osteotomies, he finally deciphered that the shortened lateral column had produced lateral rotation of the navicular on the talus that could not be simply corrected by a mechanical shift of the heel. He, therefore, realized the lateral column needed to be lengthened to medialize the heel, reduce the convexity of the medial border, and somewhat restore the natural equinus of the foot.

"In the normal foot the medial and lateral columns are about equal in length, in talipes equino-varus the lateral column is longer and in calcaneovalgus shorter than the medial column. The suggestion is that in the treatment of both deformities the length of the columns be made equal." This quote is an extract from Evans last paper entitled "Calcaneo-valgus deformity" published in August 1975.[2] Sadly, he passed away in November 1974 at the age of 64, never to witness arguably his most famous legacy.

Evolution

Before the introduction of the lateral column lengthening, treatment of the flatfoot deformity usually involved arthrodesis procedures. In Evans 1975 article, it is clear he wanted to preserve the calcaneocuboid joint. His original technique was first performed in 1959 for overcorrected talipes equinovarus, calcaneovalgus after polio, rigid flatfoot, and idiopathic calcaneovalgus. After his surgery on overcorrected club feet, he stated:

> Perhaps the most interesting single point that has emerged from this series of cases is the conversion of varus into valgus. It then became obvious that excessive shortening of the lateral border of the foot had produced an excessive lateral rotation of the navicular on the head of the talus and that the remedy was to undo the calcaneocuboid fusion and to lengthen the lateral border of the foot by inserting a wedge graft. This was tried and it produced, in varying degree,

three effects; the heel moved towards neutral, the convexity on the medial border was reduced, and the foot as a whole moved slightly into equinus.[1]

Overall, he then performed this procedure in 56 feet for a variety of conditions. He describes making an osteotomy 1.5 cm behind the joint in the anterior calcaneus but parallel to the plane of the joint. The osteotomy was then filled with ipsilateral tibial cortical bone. Non–weight-bearing in a plaster is instituted for 4 weeks with the plaster on for 4 months. Mosca and colleagues[3] modified the Evans procedure. He based his operative technique on the observation that the center of rotation for the correction is near the center of the talar head and not simply the medial calcaneal cortex; thus, the osteotomy is not a plain distracting or opening wedge osteotomy. The direction of his osteotomy was modified by directing it proximal/lateral to distal/medial in an oblique fashion; however, its starting point was 1.5 cm proximal to the calcaneocuboid joint. He then recommended filling the gap with a trapezoidal shaped tri-cortical iliac crest graft.[3]

How Does Lateral Column Lengthening Correct the Foot?

Evans' 1975 article[2] demonstrates how complex relationships and biomechanics in the foot can be theorized by simple observation: "Logic suggested that if this shape (calcaneovalgus) had been produced by excessive shortening of the lateral column (during clubfoot corrective surgery) it should be possible to improve the shape (of the foot) by lengthening the lateral column by insertion of a bone graft." Although Evans noticed that as the valgus forefoot deviation disappeared with the navicular moving medially on the talus and the heel took up a more varus posture with restoration of a more cavus midfoot on graft insertion, the exact mechanism by which lateral column lengthening corrects the foot position remains poorly understood. Radiologic evidence for improvement of foot posture was shown by Sangeorzan and associate[4] in 1993. Although a small study of only seven adults following Evans osteotomy by comparing anteroposterior and lateral projection preoperative and postoperative radiographs, they showed that lateral talocalcaneal angle improved by 6.4°, the talonavicular coverage improved by 26° and the calcaneal pitch improved by 10.8°. Their greatest angular improvement was in the talonavicular coverage, suggesting this is quite a good indicator of mid/forefoot alignment.[4] As the foot corrects, it was thought the responsible force was increased tension in the windlass mechanism akin to the Jacks hyperextension test,[3] but Horton and co-workers[5] disproved this theory by using strain gauges in the plantar fascia and actually showed that the medial fascia actually loosens by an average of 2.7 mm.[5] With improvements in computed tomography and generation of 3-dimesnional models, DuMontier and associates[6] were able to elegantly show the changes produced in the foot by performing an Evans procedure. The structure of the head of the talus affects the movement of the navicular around it. The talar head is wider in a medial-lateral direction than dorsal-plantar direction. As the lateral column is lengthened, the forefoot moves medially at the transverse tarsal joint. The navicular also moves slightly plantarward (short radius of curvature) resulting in forefoot adduction and plantarflexion and increased arch height. The navicular rotated 18.6° of adduction, 2.6° pronation, 3.4° plantarflexion, 5.6 mm medial, 0.4 mm posterior, and 1.8 mm plantar. The cuboid rotated 24.2° of adduction, 13.9° pronation, 1.9° plantarflexion, 9.4 mm medial, 2.6 mm distal, and 1.5 mm plantar. They found the calcaneum did not move into varus relative to the talus or tibia, suggesting that the significant correction of the mid and forefoot on the hindfoot gives the appearance of a calcaneovarus.[6]

Clinical Indications

Although the biomechanics of lateral column lengthening are been better understood, the clinical indications for this procedure are somewhat less clear. It is clearly mostly performed in adults for an acquired flatfoot deformity, often secondary to posterior tibialis tendon dysfunction. Once the forefoot adopts the typical flexible, abduction and pronation position clinically with subfibular impingement and calcaneovalgus the lateral column lengthening procedure may be required. It is one of a number of procedures that is utilized. Although nearly 10 years ago, Hiller and Pinney[7] surveyed orthopedic surgeons practice in the United States in dealing with a typical stage 2 adult acquired flatfoot produced some interesting findings: 38% agreed that a combined medializing calcaneal osteotomy, tibialis posterior augmentation (flexor digitorum longus or less commonly flexor hallucis longus) is required; 22% agreed that this was used in conjunction with the lateral column lengthening. Nine percent decided to perform a subtalar arthrodesis, whereas 12% performed, along with other procedures mentioned, medial column stabilization. In addition, 70% would address a tight calf complex. Although a standardized "typical case" was difficult to define, the striking feature from this study was the profound variety of performed procedures. To define a population who are likely to gain the benefit of this procedure, it is the late stage 2 category.[8] These are patients who have developed elongation and degeneration of the posterior tibial tendon with an obvious hindfoot valgus and forefoot abduction. The key is that the deformity is correctible. Subclassifying stage 2 is useful into type a, where the symptoms are primarily medial and less severe and the patient can still perform a single stance heel raise, and type b, where a more pronounced collapse has occurred with subfibular impingement. Radiographically, the patient with a significant collapse demonstrates abduction at the level of the talonavicular joint on the anteroposterior radiograph; on the lateral radiograph, there may be some midfoot sag at the talonavicular or naviculocuneiform joints. Another useful measurement can be the relationship in height between the medial cuneiform and the fifth metatarsal. It is the stage 2b patients in whom the lateral column lengthening provides a bony block to attempt to prevent later collapse of the lateral column and recurrence of deformity. To our knowledge, all cases series of lateral column lengthening procedures have been described in conjunction with combined procedures as described; thus, its efficacy alone is really unknown in vivo.

Operative Technique

Evans' early description of this technique utilized an osteotomy 1.5 cm parallel to and distal to the calcaneocuboid joint. This technique has stood the test of time, although surgeon preference dictates the graft material and fixation method (if any). As alluded to earlier, Mosca modified the osteotomy slightly, putting more emphasis on the osteotomy shape and direction to produce optimal 3-dimensional motion of the forefoot on the midfoot. Although 1.5 cm distal to the joint is an excellent starting point for the osteotomy Raines and Brage[9] performed an anatomic study to identify the safest osteotomy site. By making osteotomies at 5, 10, and 15 mm from the joint, they concluded the 10-mm interval to be the safest option to avoid both the anterior and middle facets of the subtalar joint. They also considered the position of the osteotomy to least likely damage the surrounding soft tissue structures both medially and laterally and they found that a more distal—around 5 mm—osteotomy from the calcaneocuboid joint may injure the sural nerve or peroneals, whereas placing the osteotomy more proximally—around 15 mm from the calcaneocuboid joint—may

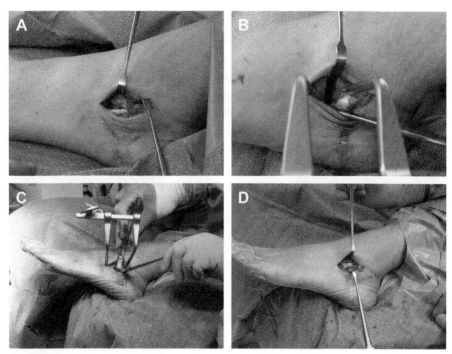

Fig. 1. (*A*) Incision exposes the anterior process of the calcaneus. (*B*) Exposure of the osteotomy using a retractor. (*C*) Insertion of the graft. (*D*) Low-profile locking plate in situ.

injure the flexor hallucis longus, flexor digitorum longus, medial plantar nerve, or tibialis posterior.[9]

Authors' Technique

This operation is usually performed under general anesthesia; however, spinal anesthesia is an alternative. The patient is positioned supine with a sandbag under the ipsilateral buttock and a rigid thigh bolster positioned to hold the hip slightly flexed, adducted, and internally rotated, with the knee slightly flexed. This aids access to the lateral side of the foot. The tourniquet is inflated and the patient prepared with an alcohol solution above the knee, including the ipsilateral iliac crest. Extremity drapes isolate the surgical field. An incision is made 5 to 7 cm in length, starting just distal to the calcaneocuboid joint going proximally in line with the superior border of the calcaneus (**Fig. 1**A). The peroneals and sural nerve are identified. The joint capsule is not violated and extensor digitorum brevis is elevated off the calcaneus. Using retraction, the anterior process is visualized and an osteotomy is made parallel to and 1 cm proximal to the joint with a small oscillating saw. Using a laminar spreader or Hintermann type retractor (see **Fig. 1**B), the osteotomy is opened and filled with (ipsilateral) tricortical iliac crest graft; alternatively, allograft femoral head can be used depending on the surgeons' preference (see **Fig. 1**C). Rigid fixation is achieved with a low-profile locking plate construct over the osteotomy (see **Fig. 1**D). Radiology is used to confirm plate position. The wound is closed with absorbable suture material. The patient is placed into a plaster cast non–weight-bearing for 4 weeks with a wound check performed at 2 weeks. After 4 weeks, the patient is examined clinically and with

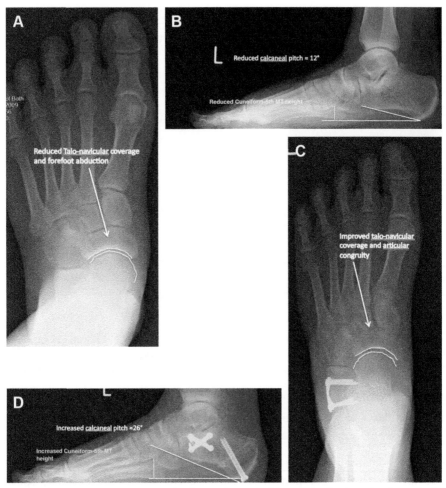

Fig. 2. (*A*) Preoperative anteroposterior foot radiograph. (*B*) Preoperative lateral radiograph. (*C*) Postoperative anteroposterior radiograph demonstrating improved talonavicular coverage. (*D*) Postoperative lateral radiograph demonstrating improved calcaneal angulation.

x-ray, and allowed to mobilize providing the osteotomy is progressing to clinical and radiologic healing. Total time with protective splinting is 10–12 weeks, with the last 6 weeks in a walking boot. Radiographs (with concomitant medializing calcaneal osteotomy) postoperatively show an improvement in calcaneal pitch angle and also a reduction in forefoot abduction with an increase in talonavicular coverage (**Fig. 2**).

The authors use a very similar technique when performing a calcaneocuboid joint distraction arthrodesis. The incision is usually extended slightly distally to adequately expose the joint. There are a number of ways to denude a joint of articular cartilage; however, the authors tend to use a fine flexible chisel to denude the bare minimum of subchondral bone ensuring the cartilage is removed without significantly altering the structural integrity of the cancellous bone. The bare surfaces are then fashioned to accommodate the flat surfaces of the bone graft on its insertion. The bone graft is then secured in the same fashion as described, with a low-profile locking plate construct.

Important Surgical Issues

Calcaneocuboid distraction arthrodesis or lengthening calcaneal osteotomy?

There is no level 1 evidence directly comparing these 2 techniques. Most studies of either technique are level 4 evidence, with a variety of other associated procedures performed and are therefore difficult to interpret.

Thomas and colleagues[8] compared the 2 techniques in 37 adult patients who had concomitant flexor digitorum longus transfers (39 feet), but only 27 feet were available for follow-up at a mean of 52 months (Evans procedure, 10 feet) and 24.7 months (arthrodesis, 17 feet). Radiographic loss of position was noted compared with initial postoperative x-rays, but the only significant difference was a small decrease in calcaneal pitch angle, that was more evident in the arthrodesis group (3.82° vs 6.44°; P = .014). Functional AOFAS (American Orthopedic Foot and Ankle Society) was not significantly different between the groups (80.9 vs 87.9). The complication rates were much higher in the arthrodesis group (7/17 in the Evans group, 16/17 in the arthrodesis group, with 14 common to both groups) despite follow-up being significantly longer in the Evans group. Of note there were 2 non-unions and 3 delayed unions in the arthrodesis group.[9]

Haeseker et al retrospectively analyzed 33 patients with adult acquired flatfeet of which 14 had distraction arthrodesis and 19 had lengthening osteotomy. Both groups in combination with medial soft tissue surgery. There was a significant difference in AOFAS (71.9 in the joint arthrodesis group at mean follow-up of 42.4 months and 84.9 in the osteotomy group at mean follow-up of 15.8 months). There was no difference between the 2 groups' radiologic parameters preoperatively or postoperatively, which was correlated with length of follow-up. The arthrodesis group reported 3 complications: a wound infection, a chronic regional pain syndrome, and a nonunion. The lengthening group reported 3 also, 1 nonunion, 1 deep venous thrombosis, and 1 wound infection.[10]

In Hiller and Pinney's survey[9] of 104 surgeons in the United States, when asked how they would treat an adult acquired flatfoot stage 2 posterior tibialis tendon dysfunction, 101 would perform a bony procedure, of which 43 would perform a lateral column lengthening; of these, roughly half would undertake an Evans and half an arthrodesis.[9] There is no consensus on which to perform, but it is the authors' opinion that joint-preserving procedures should really be advocated and an Evans-type procedure be performed when possible.

Other operative procedures are reported to attempt to give the desired effect of the more traditional methods of lateral column lengthening. Vander Griend[12] describes a Z-lengthening osteotomy of the calcaneus that incorporates a distal vertical cut 10 mm from the calcaneocuboid joint through the dorsal half of the anterior process. This is connected to a horizontal limb, full thickness through the calcaneus, and finally completed by a vertical plantar cut around the level of the peroneal tubercle. This is more technically demanding, with probably more risk to damaging medially based structures. The osteotomy is also only fixed with 1 screw that may predispose to early failure of fixation, considering the general quality of bone in this area of the calcaneus and the forces present across the osteotomy. Although the description of this technique reports only on 8 patients with no long-term follow-up it should be considered an option in the surgeons' armamentarium.[12]

Graft type

The ideal graft size has been studied extensively and recommendations have been made from both clinical and cadaveric studies. Currently, most authors advocate a graft length between 8 and 12 mm, usually 10 mm.[2,11,13-16] Corticocancellous allograft and autograft are the 2 main types used. Dolan performed a randomized, controlled trial comparing iliac crest graft with allograft for calcaneal lengthening in adults. Of the 33 feet, 18 had an allograft and 15 an autograft. All patients achieved union by 12 weeks. In the allograft group, 94% united by 8 weeks, whereas only 60% of autografts had united by 8 weeks. Two autograft cases had hip scar pain at 3 months, but is unclear whether it persisted.[17] Anecdotally, surgeons are concerned about allograft incorporation, but Mosca[3] also achieved 100% union in 24 cases with allograft and 7 with autograft use in modified Evans procedures, albeit in children. Grier and Walling[18] compared tricortical allograft and autograft both supplemented with platelet-rich plasma in adults in both joint arthrodesis and Evans procedures; they achieved 94% union with allograft and 70% with autograft. Philbin and co-workers[19] achieved 96% union in 28 feet undergoing lengthening with fresh-frozen tricortical grafts. Templin and associates[20] report 97% union in 30 pediatric cases of lengthenings. Other studies report mainly on the use of iliac crest autograft and union rates vary from 80% to 100% in both calcaneocuboid arthrodesis and Evans-type procedures.[10,20-24]

Iliac crest donor site morbidity can potentially be a site of morbidity; however, in foot surgery the donor volume requirements are usually low, necessitating only a small incision with minimal resection. Morbidity reported varies from 2.4% up to 31% suffering from chronic pain after 2 years.[25-27]

Graft collapse and loss of correction can potentially be a source of concern after lateral column lengthening procedures, but clinical correlation can be difficult. In a large pediatric, series Danko and colleagues[28] found 17 of 58 of calcaneocuboid joint arthrodesis allografts and 3 of 3 autografts collapsed, but neither allograft nor autograft used in their Evans procedures collapsed.[28] They suggested lateral column lengthening through the anterior process of the calcaneus is a more durable option. Conti and Wong[29] also experienced graft collapse in 16% of distraction arthrodeses. Five out of 6 were fixed with a K-wire and 1 with an H-plate. It is likely that lack of stability with wire fixation contributed to failure and ultimately collapse.[29] Kimball and associates[30] studied the properties of screw and plate fixation in lateral column lengthening and discovered that nearly 3 times the force was required to create a 1-mm graft–host interface with plate fixation. Collapse of allograft may also be due to the mechanical properties of the material that may be adversely affected by the method of sterilization and storage.[31] Fresh-frozen grafts tend to have least impact on strength although biomechanical studies have shown that irradiating or freeze drying bone does not significantly reduce ultimate tensile stress/strain compared with controls.[32] The authors were unable to uncover any objective clinical evidence for the use of synthetic materials specific to lateral column lengthening procedures as a graft in either calcaneocuboid distraction arthrodesis or anterior process lengthenings; however, current research into the use of synthetic materials in foot and ankle arthrodesis models is showing some promising results. Digiovanni and co-workers[33] performed a randomized, controlled trial with the recombinant form of platelet-derived growth factor, which was utilized as a bone graft substitute material in all hindfoot fusion procedures. They randomized this material with autologous bone graft harvest. At 36 weeks, fusion rates were available in 18 patients, with 10 of 13 (72%) synthetic grafts and 3 of 6 (50%) autologous grafts achieving fusion. Although one may consider these are relatively low fusion rates, the results suggest synthetic grafts may be a suitable alternative to autograft, with no donor site morbidity.[33]

Degenerative joint disease

Lateral column lengthening through the calcaneocuboid joint is an alternative to joint-preserving surgery. Evans suggested preserving the joint through his osteotomy; however, studies have shown that the contact pressure generated across the calcaneocuboid joint after lengthening may actually rise, raising concerns that this may predispose to early degenerative change. Cooper and colleagues[34] performed measurement of pressures across the calcaneocuboid joint during lengthening procedures in 8 fresh frozen, below-the-knee amputation specimens and discovered that the pressure increase across the joint were proportional to the degree of lengthening undertaken. They recorded pressures at 0, 5, and 10 mm of lengthening. They did, however, perform the osteotomy at 15 mm proximal to the joint, and not at 10 mm as often recommended. More recently, Iaquinto and Wayne[16] performed a computed tomography cadaveric study to determine the effects of surgical correction of the adult acquired flatfoot. An Evans procedure was modeled by creating an osteotomy 10 mm proximal to the calcaneocuboid joint with 10 mm of opening; a distraction arthrodesis was performed by denuding articular cartilage and inserting a 10-mm wedge. They found that joint contact pressures were increased from baseline levels after Evans procedures by 111%. The addition of a medializing calcaneal osteotomy reduced this pressure increase to 93%.[16] Momberger and associate,[35] on the other hand, simulated flatfoot deformities in cadaveric specimens and concluded that, although pressure across the calcaneocuboid joint is higher than normal in planovalgus feet, there was no significant rise in pressure after lateral column lengthening of these feet. Nevertheless, concerns that degenerative changes develop in the calcaneocuboid joint in longer term follow-up studies[36,37] have led some surgeons opting for primary distraction arthrodesis of the calcaneocuboid joint.[11,24] This loss of motion at the calcaneocuboid joint has been shown to have minimal overall effect on the motion of the hindfoot complex.[38,39] Deland also showed that 1-cm lateral column lengthening after calcaneocuboid joint arthrodesis maintained 48% of talonavicular and 70% of subtalar movement. Inversion at the talonavicular joint was 66% of normal and subtalar inversion was 88% of normal.[40]

Lateral foot pain

Continued lateral foot discomfort can be an issue postoperatively after any lateral column lengthening procedure. Although the operation can correct the abduction of the forefoot, it may not reliably correct the supination deformity in the axial plane. This can subsequently cause the patient to overload the lateral border on weight bearing, which can be significantly distressing to the patient. As a result of this column overload, reports of stress fractures to the base of the fifth metatarsal have emerged.[10,41] Tien and colleagues[13] hypothesized that, by performing a distraction arthrodesis at the level of the Chopart joint, it would allow the surgeon more freedom to rotate the forefoot on the midfoot, thus potentially reducing the plantar pressures in comparison with a more proximally based osteotomy for an Evans-type procedure. They found, however, that the plantar pressure increases under the fifth metatarsal head were statistically greater for the distraction arthrodeses procedure than the Evans-type procedure.[13] This study to some degree echoed the findings of Thomas and associates,[11] in a clinical study previously mentioned. Among 34 feet, 17 underwent Evans procedures and 17 calcaneocuboid joint fusions. In the fusion group, 3 had graft stress fractures, 1 had a fifth metatarsal fracture, and 3 had "residual supination" deformities. All of these complications may quite easily either result in or lead to lateral foot overload. It is likely that the effect of forefoot overload may be related to the degree of correction achieved at the osteotomy or arthrodesis site. It has been suggested that by carefully templating the correction to be achieved intraoperatively by using trial metal wedges in the osteotomy site during an Evans-type procedure before introduction of the graft can reduce the incidence of postoperative plantar lateral foot pain. Ellis and co-workers[14] developed the simple idea of intraoperative metal wedge templates to subjectively measure the correction of the talonavicular abduction and degree of forefoot stiffness in eversion after the insertion of the wedge into the osteotomy site. Before the use of trial wedges intraoperatively, the incidence of patient reported lateral foot pain was 14.7%; after the introduction of the wedges, the incidence decreased to 6.3% ($P = .084$). Although not a significant reduction in reported pain, they did find the revision rates were significantly reduced after use of trial wedges (from 12.8% to 3.7%; $P = .03$). Their average graft length was 6.8 mm (range, 4–10).[14] It is possible, therefore, by simply reducing the length of the graft, to potentially reduce the effect of lateral foot overload. It has also been suggested that the surgeon should, as well as reducing the graft length, attempt to plantarflex and adduct at the osteotomy site by shaping the graft like a trapezoid Chopart joint.[42] This is similar to the Mosca trapezoidal wedge,[3] which is a wedge with a lateral border 10 to 12 mm long and a medial border of 4 to 6 mm (Mosca does not describe a plantar-flexing effect of the graft). After internal fixation of the lateral column, patients can sometimes complain of prominent metalwork, especially if the foot is not fully corrected. Delayed metalwork removal is necessary in up to 30% of cases,[17,19,23,29,41] and this should be remembered when planning surgical fixation. Taking this into account, the authors recommend the use of lower profile locking plates that may reduce the risk of structural irritation and of later hardware removal.

SUMMARY

Lateral column lengthening procedures, either an Evans-type procedure or a calcaneocuboid distraction arthrodesis, clearly have a role to play in the management of a pes planovalgus foot deformity, as is evident from clinical outcome studies. Despite an abundance of literature intricately detailing the biomechanical effects of different operative procedures on the hindfoot, there is no clear consensus as to the best procedure or procedures to perform for a flexible pes planovalgus foot deformity. There is, therefore, no single solution to this problem; the surgeon must treat each patient as an individual and choose the procedure that will work best in their hands for any given foot pathology they are presented with. The surgeon must also be aware that to improve the kinematics of a planovalgus foot deformity, one may often have to perform multiple procedures and not a lateral column lengthening in isolation.

REFERENCES

1. Evans D. Relapsed club foot. J Bone Joint Surg Br 1961;43B:722–33.
2. Evans D. Calcaneo-valgus deformity. J Bone Joint Surg Br 1975;57:270–8.
3. Mosca VS. Calcaneal lengthening for valgus deformity of the hindfoot. Results in children who had severe, symptomatic flatfoot and skewfoot. J Bone Joint Surg Am 1995;77:500–12.
4. Sangeorzan BJ, Mosca V, Hansen ST. Effect of calcaneal lengthening on relationships among the hindfoot, midfoot, and forefoot. Foot Ankle 1993;14:136–41.

5. Horton GA, Myerson MS, Parks BG, et al. Effect of calcaneal osteotomy and lateral column lengthening on the plantar fascia: a biomechanical investigation. Foot Ankle Int 1998;19:370–3.

6. Dumontier TA, Falicov A, Mosca V, et al. Calcaneal lengthening: investigation of deformity correction in a cadaver flatfoot model. Foot Ankle Int 2005;26: 166–70.

7. Hiller L, Pinney SJ. Surgical treatment of acquired flatfoot deformity: what is the state of practice among academic foot and ankle surgeons in 2002? Foot Ankle Int 2003;24:701–5.

8. Johnson KA, Strom DE. Tibialis posterior tendon dysfunction. Clin Orthop Relat Res 1989;196-206.

9. Raines RA, Brage ME. Evans osteotomy in the adult foot: an anatomic study of structures at risk. Foot Ankle Int 1998;19:743–7.

10. Haeseker GA, Mureau MA, Faber FW. Lateral column lengthening for acquired adult flatfoot deformity caused by posterior tibial tendon dysfunction stage II: a retrospective comparison of calcaneus osteotomy with calcaneocuboid distraction arthrodesis. J Foot Ankle Surg 2010;49:380–4.

11. Thomas RL, Wells BC, Garrison RL, et al. Preliminary results comparing two methods of lateral column lengthening. Foot Ankle Int 2001;22:107–19.

12. Vander Griend R. Lateral column lengthening using a "Z" osteotomy of the calcaneus. Techniques in Foot and Ankle Surgery 2008;7:257–63.

13. Tien TR, Parks BG, Guyton GP. Plantar pressures in the forefoot after lateral column lengthening: a cadaver study comparing the Evans osteotomy and calcaneocuboid fusion. Foot Ankle Int 2005;26:520–5.

14. Ellis, SJ, Williams BR, Garg R, et al. Incidence of plantar lateral foot pain before and after the use of trial metal wedges in lateral column lengthening. Foot Ankle Int 2011;32:665–73.

15. Pomeroy GC, Pike RH, Beals TC, et al. Acquired flatfoot in adults due to dysfunction of the posterior tibial tendon. J Bone Joint Surg Am 1999;81:1173–82.

16. Iaquinto JM, Wayne JS. Effects of surgical correction for the treatment of adult acquired flatfoot deformity: a computational investigation. J Orthop Res 2011;29: 1047–54.

17. Dolan CM, Henning JA, Anderson JG, et al. Randomized prospective study comparing tri-cortical iliac crest autograft to allograft in the lateral column lengthening component for operative correction of adult acquired flatfoot deformity. Foot Ankle Int 2007;28:8–12.

18. Grier KM, Walling AK. The use of tricortical autograft versus allograft in lateral column lengthening for adult acquired flatfoot deformity: an analysis of union rates and complications. Foot Ankle Int 2010;31:760–9.

19. Philbin TM, Pokabla C, Berlet GC. Lateral column lengthening using allograft interposition and cervical plate fixation. Foot Ankle Spec 2008;1:288–96.

20. Templin D, Jones K, Weiner DS. The incorporation of allogeneic and autogenous bone graft in healing of lateral column lengthening of the calcaneus. J Foot Ankle Surg 2008;47:283–7.

21. Oh I, Williams BR, Ellis SJ, et al. Reconstruction of the symptomatic idiopathic flatfoot in adolescents and young adults. Foot Ankle Int 2011;32:225–32.

22. Hintermann B, Valderrabano V, Kundert HP. Lengthening of the lateral column and reconstruction of the medial soft tissue for treatment of acquired flatfoot deformity associated with insufficiency of the posterior tibial tendon. Foot Ankle Int 1999;20: 622–9.

23. Bolt PM, Coy S, Toolan BC. A comparison of lateral column lengthening and medial translational osteotomy of the calcaneus for the reconstruction of adult acquired flatfoot. Foot Ankle Int 2007;28:1115–23.

24. Toolan BC, Sangeorzan BJ, Hansen ST. Complex reconstruction for the treatment of dorsolateral peritalar subluxation of the foot. Early results after distraction arthrodesis of the calcaneocuboid joint in conjunction with stabilization of, and transfer of the flexor digitorum longus tendon to, the midfoot to treat acquired pes planovalgus in adults. J Bone Joint Surg Am 1999;81:1545–60.

25. Silber JS, Anderson DG, Daffner SD, et al. Donor site morbidity after anterior iliac crest bone harvest for single-level anterior cervical discectomy and fusion. Spine (Phila Pa 1976) 2003;28:134-9.

26. Sasso RC, LeHuec JC, Shaffrey C, et al. Iliac crest bone graft donor site pain after anterior lumbar interbody fusion: a prospective patient satisfaction outcome assessment. J Spinal Disord Tech 2005;18(Suppl):S77–81.

27. Schulhofer SD, Oloff LM. Iliac crest donor site morbidity in foot and ankle surgery. J Foot Ankle Surg 1997;36:155–8.

28. Danko AM, Allen B, Pugh L, et al. Early graft failure in lateral column lengthening. J Pediatr Orthop 2004;24:716–20.

29. Conti SF, Wong YS. Osteolysis of structural autograft after calcaneocuboid distraction arthrodesis for stage II posterior tibial tendon dysfunction. Foot Ankle Int 2002;23:521–9.

30. Kimball HL, Aronow MS, Sullivan RJ, et al. Biomechanical evaluation of calcaneocuboid distraction arthrodesis: a cadaver study of two different fixation methods. Foot Ankle Int 2000;21:845–8.

31. Pelker RR, Friedlaender GE, Markham TC. Biomechanical properties of bone allografts. Clin Orthop Relat Res 1983;(174):54-7.

32. Mikhael MM, Huddleston PM, Zobitz ME, et al. Mechanical strength of bone allografts subjected to chemical sterilization and other terminal processing methods. J Biomech 2008;41:2816–20.

33. Digiovanni CW, Baumhauer J, Lin SS, et al. Prospective, randomized, multi-center feasibility trial of rhPDGF-BB versus autologous bone graft in a foot and ankle fusion model. Foot Ankle Int 2011;32:344–54.

34. Cooper PS, Nowak MD, Shaer J. Calcaneocuboid joint pressures with lateral column lengthening (Evans) procedure. Foot Ankle Int 1997;18:199–205.

35. Momberger N, Morgan JM, Bachus KN, et al. Calcaneocuboid joint pressure after lateral column lengthening in a cadaveric planovalgus deformity model. Foot Ankle Int 2000;21:730–5.

36. Phillips GE. A review of elongation of os calcis for flat feet. J Bone Joint Surg Br 1983;65:15–8.

37. Moseir-LaClair S, Pomeroy G, Manoli A. Intermediate follow-up on the double osteotomy and tendon transfer procedure for stage II posterior tibial tendon insufficiency. Foot Ankle Int 2001;22:283–91.

38. Astion DJ, Deland JT, Otis JC, et al. Motion of the hindfoot after simulated arthrodesis. J Bone Joint Surg Am 1997;79:241–6.

39. Wülker N, Stukenborg C, Savory KM, et al. Hindfoot motion after isolated and combined arthrodeses: measurements in anatomic specimens. Foot Ankle Int 2000;21:921–7.

40. O'Malley MJ, Deland JT, Lee KT. Selective hindfoot arthrodesis for the treatment of adult acquired flatfoot deformity: an in vitro study. Foot Ankle Int 1995;16:411–7.

41. Chi TD, Toolan BC, Sangeorzan BJ, et al. The lateral column lengthening and medial column stabilization procedures. Clin Orthop Relat Res 1999;81–90.

42. Neufeld SK, Myerson MS. Complications of surgical treatments for adult flatfoot deformities. Foot Ankle Clin 2001;6:179–91.

Is There a Role for Subtalar Arthroereisis in the Management of Adult Acquired Flatfoot?

Pablo Fernández de Retana, MD[a],*, Fernando Álvarez, MD[b],
Gustavo Bacca, MD[b]

KEYWORDS

- Adult acquired • Arthroereisis • Pes planovalgus • Subtalar implant
- Subtalar joint

KEY POINTS

- Subtalar arthroereisis is 1 treatment option for stage IIA posterior tibial tendon dysfunction, as an alternative to calcaneal medializing osteotomy.
- Subtalar arthroereisis, often combined with Achilles tendon lengthening, is a simple and effective way to treat flexible flatfoot in adults.
- The most common complication is pain in sinus tarsi that usually disappears after removal of implant. Midterm results are good and it does not hinder other treatments in the future.

Adult acquired flatfoot is a common problem for foot and ankle surgeons. The incidence is increasing and it is becoming more widely known among orthopedic surgeons in the last years. The main cause is rupture of posterior tibial tendon (PTT). The morphologic characteristics of this condition are heel valgus and flattening of the medial longitudinal arch. Other characteristics are usually observed, such as supination and abduction of the forefoot and tightening of the Achilles tendon. The deformity is progressive and patients describe "sinking" of their foot. There is no spontaneous correction with time and many patients become symptomatic. Treatment is required when there is progression of deformity and/or pain. Conservative treatment includes supportive footwear and ankle orthosis.[1] The natural evolution of adult flatfoot and failure to treat this condition could lead to persistent pain in the hindfoot, hallux valgus, degenerative arthritis, metatarsalgia, and knee or low back pain.

[a] Orthopaedic Surgery Department, Hospital San Rafael, Passeig Vall d'Hebron 107-117, 08035 Barcelona, Spain; [b] Foot and Ankle Unit, Orthopaedic Surgery Department, Hospital San Rafael, Passeig Vall d'Hebron 107-117, 08035 Barcelona, Spain
* Corresponding author.
E-mail address: pfernan@hsrafael.es

Foot Ankle Clin N Am 17 (2012) 271–281
http://dx.doi.org/10.1016/j.fcl.2012.03.006
1083-7515/12/$ – see front matter © 2012 Elsevier Inc. All rights reserved.

Surgery is commonly indicated in adult flatfeet. Flexible flatfoot should be treated preferably with extra-articular procedures. There are different surgical options: Tendon transfers, osteotomies, and subtalar joint motion blocking procedures. Shortening of the gastrocnemius or the Achilles tendon is very common in flatfoot. Often, it is necessary to lengthen these structures. The final decision is usually based on the clinical and radiographic assessment of the patient on an individual basis and the surgeon's preferences. Chambers[2] in 1946 was the first to introduce the idea of restricting subtalar joint motion with an autologous bone block filling the sinus tarsi. In 1952, Grice[3] observed that extra-articular subtalar arthrodesis with cortical graft for flatfoot deformity in children had several problems, such as development of degenerative arthritis in adjacent joints and inability of the hindfoot to adapt to uneven surfaces. Haraldsson[4] and Lelievre[5] pointed out that the most important was to block the sinus tarsi restricting subtalar motion while avoiding arthrodesis. Since then, the term arthroereisis (Latin: *artro* = joint; *-ereisis* = support or prop up) is used to describe the limitation of subtalar motion.[5] Viladot and co-workers[6] presented their experience treating PTT dysfunction stage II with arthroereisis.

SUBTALAR ARTHROEREISIS WITH SINUS TARSI IMPLANT

Arthroereisis has been used predominantly to treat flatfeet in the pediatric population.[7,8] Many arthroereisis procedures have been described to limit subtalar joint motion and to improve position. Lelievre[5] in 1970 introduced the term lateral arthroereisis using a temporary staple across the subtalar joint. In 1977, Subotnick[9] was the first to describe a sinus tarsi implant. He used a block of silicone elastamer. Smith and Millar[10] used a polyethylene screw in sinus tarsi (STA peg, Dow Corning Wright, Midland, MI, USA) and reported a 96% success rate in children. Viladot[11] reported the use of a silicon implant with a cup shape, obtaining 99% good results in 234 children. Presently, Silicon implants are not usually used and have been replaced with troncoconical implants like Kalix (New Deal, Lyon, France) and MBA (Kinitekos Medical, Carlsbad, CA, USA). Zaret and Myerson[7] reported 23 children with flexible flatfoot treated with MBA implants.[7] They reported postoperative sinus tarsi pain in 18% of patients that improved with rest and corticosteroid injection. Two children required implant removal at a mean of 9 months after surgery. Subtalar joint range of motion increased after implant removal. They observed an interesting phenomenon: Removal of the implant was not associated with a reversal of the foot structure.

Vogler[12] classified sinus tarsi implants into 3 types based on their biomechanical properties: Self-locking wedge, axis-altering implant, and impact-blocking device.[12] The majority of sinus tarsi implants are self-locking wedges. All sinus tarsi devices restrict hindfoot valgus and the calcaneus is vertically orientated beneath the ankle joint.[8] The talus is dorsiflexed and externally deviated. Talonavicular subluxation and forefoot abduction are corrected.

Indications

According to Johnson and Strom,[13] PTT dysfunction is classified in 3 stages. Stage I PTT has degenerative changes, but no deformity. Stage II is a flexible flatfoot. In the beginning, the hindfoot is in valgus and progresses to abduction and supination in the forefoot. Stage III is a rigid deformity. Myerson[14] described stage IV when the ankle joint is affected. Recently, a refined classification system has been proposed that takes into account forefoot supination, forefoot abduction, and medial column instability.[15] Stage II has been subclassified in A, B, and C substages. There is a valgus deformity in substage A, abduction in substage B, and medial column stability in substage C.

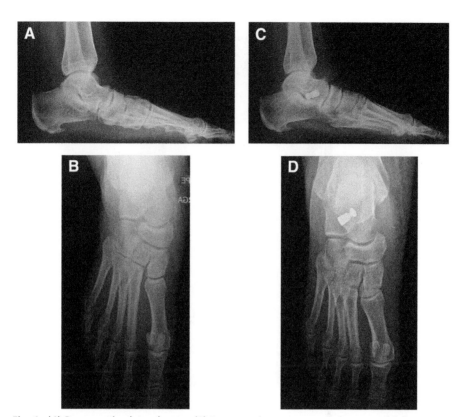

Fig. 1. (A) Preoperative lateral x-ray. (B) Preoperative anteroposterior x-ray. (C) Postoperative lateral x-ray with Kalix endorthesis. The forefoot is in slight supination. (D) Postoperative anteroposterior x-ray with Kalix in supple adduction.

Surgery is indicated for symptomatic flatfoot stage II, which persists despite nonsurgical treatment or when progression of deformity is observed. Tenosynovectomy is not recommended for stage II disease.[16] Surgical options are osteotomies, medial column arthrodesis, tendon transfers, and sinus tarsi implants. Sinus tarsi implants are useful for correcting valgus (substage A). Forefoot abduction (substage B and C) will not be corrected with sinus tarsi implant, even though temporarily some forefoot adduction and supination is observed after arthroereisis (**Fig. 1**).

Flexor digitorum longus (FDL) transfer has become a mainstay for soft-tissue procedures in patients with stage II PTT dysfunction.[14,17] Biomechanical analysis shows no change in arch alignment or height with this procedure alone.[18] When performed alone, it fails to restore normal biomechanics of the foot.[14] It has long been recognized that the spring ligament is essential in the foot structure.[19] It should be sutured or replaced when it is torn. An osteotomy should be used to correct deformity in the long term. Medial displacement calcaneal osteotomy (MDCO) and FDL tendon transfer is commonly accepted for treatment in stage IIA (valgus deformity). Sinus tarsi implant and FDL transfer has the same indication as MDCO and FDL transfer. The advantages of arthroereisis compared with MDCO are that is easy and quick to perform, less immobilization is required, there is no risk of nonunion, and it avoids

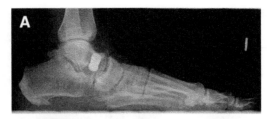

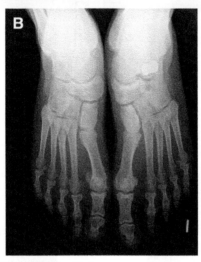

Fig. 2. (*A, B*) Loss of position of the implant.

medial neurovascular structures injuries, troughing, and malunion. It has been demonstrated that the use of a subtalar arthroereisis returns substantially deforming forces and moments of the flatfoot back toward the values experienced in a normal foot.[20] The disadvantages of arthroereisis are a high percentage of implant intolerance (around 30% in our experience) and limitation of subtalar motion. There are no controlled trial studies comparing these techniques and the level of scientific evidence is low.

Complications

Complications may be divided into general and implant specific.[8] General complications include persistent sinus tarsi pain, malposition, overcorrection, undercorrection, wrong implant size, and loss of position (**Fig. 2**).[8] The most common complication is intolerance of the implant owing to pain. Saxena and Nguyen[21] indicated that the implants must be designed and shaped to fit adequately the configuration of the tarsal sinus tarsi. Overcorrection is a cause of pain in sinus tarsi and implant removal has been recommended with good results.[22] Debris from wear, foreign body reaction, implant degradation, and implant fracture are implant-specific complications.[8] Arthritis, synovitis, implant fracture, and implant loosening have been reported with the STA-peg implant.[10] There are case reports of intraosseous cysts within the talus,[23] osteonecrosis of the talus,[24] peroneal muscle spasms, and small fracture of the calcaneus.[25] The authors have observed a case with complex regional pain syndrome type I in a patient with a sinus implant (**Fig. 3**).

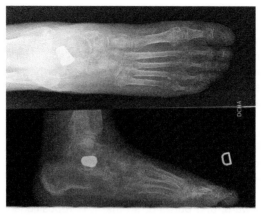

Fig. 3. Complex regional pain syndrome type I after Sinus implant.

Wound complications can occur with surgical incisions. Predisposing factors for development of these complications include tissue quality, lack of subcutaneous tissue around approaches, and postoperative swelling.[26]

Operative Technique

The authors usually perform foot surgery under block anesthesia in adults. The patient is placed in a supine position with a pillow under the ipsilateral buttock to avoid excessive external rotation of the foot and facilitate approach to the sinus tarsi. A pneumatic tourniquet is applied at the thigh and the surgical field is prepared leaving the leg exposed.

In most cases, the first step of the operation is the lengthening of the Achilles tendon. To evaluate whether this tendon is retracted, the authors hold the foot with the hindfoot in neutral position and the knee completely extended. After that, the authors passively dorsiflex the foot. If the authors cannot achieve 10° of dorsiflexion, the authors consider that the Achilles tendon is retracted and it needs to be lengthened. This helps in correcting valgus of the calcaneus and implanting the endorthesis. The authors recommend percutaneous lengthening. Two 5-mm-long incisions are performed on the lateral border of the tendon (at 2 and 6 cm from its insertion in the calcaneus) and one 5-mm-long incision on the medial border (4 cm from the insertion). Through each incision, the tendon is divided transversely approximately half of its width. The foot is dorsiflexed so that the tendon is lengthened until about 15° of dorsiflexion is obtained while the knee is extended.

FDL transfer is made through a medial incision along the entire length of the PTT. The sheath of the PTT is opened and the tendon is inspected. A tenodesis is recommended between the PTT and FDL when the PTT is healthy. FDL transfer is performed if the PTT is in poor condition. The spring ligament should be repaired if there is a disruption. The FDL is passed through the hole in the navicular from plantar to dorsal.[14] The tendon is sutured after insertion of sinus tarsi implant. It is important that the implant (final or trial implant) is inserted before completing the tendon transfer. If it is not done this way, the tension of the tendon will probably be wrong and the transfer will fail.

For implantation of the arthroereisis plug, a slightly curved 2-cm skin incision is made on the lateral side of the hindfoot centered over the sinus tarsi, just anterior to the tip of the lateral malleolus. Care must be taken not to damage the peroneal tendons, the sural nerve, and the intermediate dorsal cutaneous nerve (a branch of the superficial peroneal nerve). A direct approach to the sinus tarsi is obtained. The sinus tarsi is debrided removing its contents: fatty tissue with abundant nerve endings. This is important to eliminate the irritating stimuli of the endorthesis in the sinus, which could originate the contracture of the peroneal tendons. The powerful interosseous talocalcaneal ligament must not be damaged, because it is an important hindfoot stabilizer.

The next step consists of restoration of the foot arch and correction of calcaneous valgus deviation. This is achieved using a blunt lever, which is introduced through the sinus tarsi and under the neck of the talus. The correcting procedure is performed: The lever is pushed distally, so that the hindfoot is supinated. At the same time, the assistant pronates the forefoot. The aim of this procedure is to move the head of the talus upward, backward, and outward, so that it is repositioned in its physiologic position and hindfoot pronation is corrected. It is important to bear in mind that, in flatfoot, the talus has slipped forward, downward, and inward.

To conserve the correction obtained, an endorthesis is inserted in the sinus tarsi. First, the trial implants (with increasing diameters) are inserted until the appropriate implant size is determined. The authors choose the smallest implant that corrects the deformity and remains stable in the sinus tarsi while moving the subtalar joint. It is advisable to check the correct position of the trial implant with fluoroscopy. The authors consider that the implant is in the correct position when the lateral edge of the implant is aligned with the lateral border of the talus. Then, the definitive endorthesis is implanted, the same size as the trial implant. The FDL is sutured in a slight inversion permitting plantigrade position simulating weight bearing. Hemostasia is done after taking off Esmarch. Closure of the wound is performed in a routine fashion and a below-the-knee compression cast is applied. The whole procedure does not take more than 40 to 50 minutes. If necessary, additional procedures can be associated, including removal of accessory navicular bone, removal of tarsal coalition, and peroneal tendon lengthening.

Postoperative management

A below-the-knee walking cast is applied and sutures are removed 2 to 3 weeks postoperatively. A walker is placed when the skin has healed and weight-bearing is allowed. If there is pain with weight-bearing, the patient should avoid weight-bearing. The walker is removed 6 weeks after surgery if there is no pain with weight-bearing. The patient is advised to wear rigid orthopedic insoles for 6 months to support the correction.

Endorthesis

Since 1998, the authors have been using the Kalix endorthesis (Newdeal SA, Vienne, France) for child and adult flatfoot surgical treatment (**Fig. 4**). This implant consists of a metal cone trunk, which is introduced into another polyethylene cone trunk that expands. It is manufactured with biocompatible materials: Titanium and high-density polyethylene. Its conical shape fits well into the sinus tarsi and the lateral fins prevent the implant from moving out of the sinus tarsi. In 2009, the authors started using the Sinus implant (**Fig. 5**). It is a troncoconical device that can be screwed into the sinus tarsi. Both implants can be visualized radiographically owing to their metallic component.

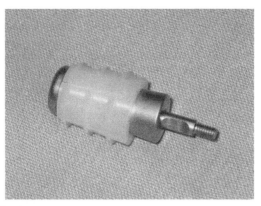

Fig. 4. Kalix endorthesis.

RESULTS

Subtalar arthroereisis has proved to yield good mid to long-term results in children.[9-11,27] However, there is little scientific evidence that proves its usefulness in adults with acquired flatfoot deformity.[7] Lelievre[5] treated flatfeet in children and adults inserting a bone graft into the sinus tarsi reporting a 90% success rate. Maxwell and associates[28] described the use of the Maxwell-Brancheau arthroereisis for the correction of PTT dysfunction having successful outcomes. Zaret and Myerson[7] reported on 12 adults treated with the MBA prosthesis. Good clinical and radiographic results were obtained, although 2 patients required removal of the prosthesis owing to persistent sinus tarsi pain; no recurrence of the deformity was observed in these patients after prosthesis removal. Viladot and colleagues[6] studied 19 patients with stage II PTT dysfunction treated with Kalix implant and tendon repair. They excluded overweight patients, those who had previous surgery, and neuropathic and osteoarthritic foot. American Orthopedic Foot and Ankle Society (AOFAS) score improved from 47.2 to 81.6 at follow-up. Only 2 patients were dissatisfied. Two patients required implant removal. Needleman[29] reported his results on 28 feet with flatfoot deformities in adult patients (≥18 years old) using an MBA implant. He

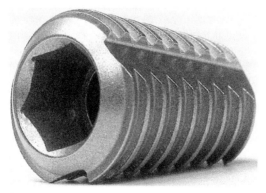

Fig. 5. Sinus implant.

included neurologic flatfoot. The exclusion criteria included infection, rigid flatfoot, evidence of osteoarthritis, and previous hindfoot surgery. Excessive weight did not affect inclusion in this study. AOFAS score improved from 52 to 87 points, and 78% of patients were satisfied with the result. Four patients (5 feet; 18%) said that they would not have the surgery again. The MBA implant was removed from 11 of 28 feet (39%) because of postoperative sinus tarsi pain.

More recently, Adelman and co-workers[30] reported their results on 10 patients with symptomatic stage IIB PTT dysfunction treated by endoscopic gastrocnemius recession, subtalar arthroereisis with the MBA implant and FDL tendon transfer to tarsal navicular. All patients showed significant improvement of radiologic measurements. Four patients (40%) referred pain at sinus tarsi but only 1 patient required implant removal. The authors conclude that this surgical combination provides satisfactory correction of stage II PTT dysfunction.

Arthroereisis has been used for treatment in children with talocalcaneal coalition owing to bad results after interposition. The results were encouraging.[31] The use in adults needs to be determined with more studies.

DISCUSSION

Acquired flexible flatfoot in adults is a common condition that requires surgery in most cases. If they fulfill the inclusion criteria mentioned, surgical treatment is indicated. Numerous treatment options have been proposed and, probably, there is not a single treatment that is appropriate for every patient. The operative procedure most frequently used to treat adult flatfoot secondary to stage II PTT dysfunction consists of MDCO and FDL transfer. This technique has proven to be effective for this condition, although calcaneal osteotomies are not free from complications. Myerson and colleagues[32] published good results in 129 patients, but with these complications directly or indirectly related to the calcaneal osteotomy: One progressive hindfoot valgus deformity, 2 varus malunion of the osteotomy, 3 sural neuritis, and 5 numbness in the distribution of the medial plantar nerve. Greene and associates[33] studied the relationship between the MDCO and the medial neurovascular structures in 22 cadaver specimens. They found that the osteotomy site was crossed by an average of 4 neurovascular structures, most of them branches of the lateral plantar nerve and the posterior tibial artery.

Subtalar arthroereisis is an alternative to calcaneal osteotomy in the treatment of stage II PTT dysfunction, particularly in stage IIA, where valgus hindfoot is the main deformity. These are the advantages of subtalar arthroereisis compared with MDCO: It is easy and quick to perform; it is a less invasive procedure; there is no risk of nonunion or malunion; there is no risk of damaging medial neurovascular structures and the sural nerve; and it requires less immobilization time and less non–weight-bearing time after surgery (shorter recovery time). Subtalar arthroereisis has a greater potential of hindfoot valgus correction than calcaneal osteotomy: The limit for calcaneal displacement is one third of its width approximately, whereas greater valgus correction can be achieved with arthroereisis using increasing implant sizes. Finally, subtalar arthroereisis provides a 3-dimensional correction of the flatfoot deformity by repositioning the talus in its physiologic position, preventing it from slipping forward, inward, and downward. It is not so clear that MDCO provides this type of correction.

There are also disadvantages of subtalar arthroereisis: It limits subtalar motion, although it is not completely blocked. The rate of pain at sinus tarsi is high (10%–40% of patients); this pain may be temporary and may require implant removal. Another

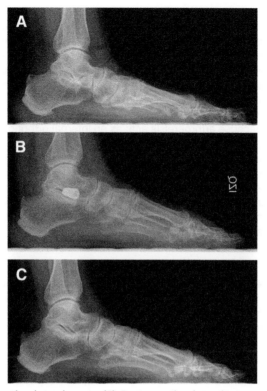

Fig. 6. (A) Preoperative lateral x-ray. (B) Postoperative lateral x-ray with Sinus subtalar arthroereisis. (C) Lateral x-ray after Sinus implant removal. The correction continues after removal.

disadvantage of arthroereisis is that most implants in the market are more expensive than the 1 or 2 screws needed for calcaneal osteotomy.

Calcaneal osteotomy and subtalar arthroereisis can be performed combined on the same patient. Schon[34] performs the MDCO first and, if he cannot achieve proper heel position with the osteotomy, he performs a subtalar arthroereisis through a different approach to gain more heel valgus correction.[34] Finally, he repairs the PTT. The authors prefer to start with the arthroereisis because, if more correction is needed, the authors use a bigger size implant and, in most cases, the calcaneal osteotomy is not needed. In any case, the fact is that both techniques can be associated if needed. Bruyn and colleagues[35] had good results using a combination of Evans calcaneal osteotomy and STA-arthroereisis. They reported 25 symptomatic severe flexible pes valgo planus treated with a combined operative technique and patients were 100% satisfied or very satisfied. The authors do not recommend combining subtalar arthroereisis with a calcaneal lengthening osteotomy. In this situation, the osteotomy is performed very close to the implant site and implant stability may be at risk.

Only minor complications have been reported with subtalar arthroereisis in adults. Sinus tarsi pain is the most frequent complication.[6-8,30,33] Different causes could explain sinus tarsi pain: Impingement of the implant against the posterior subtalar facet and irritation of the nerve ends at the sinus tarsi caused by the prosthesis or implantation of an oversized prosthesis. When this complication develops, it can be managed in different ways: Immobilization in a brace for several weeks, physiotherapy, or corticosteroid injections into the sinus tarsi. These treatments solve the problem in most, but not all, patients. When pain persists, removal of the implant is indicated. The question is: Can implant removal cause a relapse of the deformity? Almost all the literature available on subtalar arthroereisis in children and adults agrees that the possibility of recurrence is very low after implant removal. It is also our experience that implant removal usually eliminates sinus tarsi pain without clinical or radiologic recurrence of the flatfoot (**Fig. 6**). The authors think that this phenomenon can be explained because arthroereisis acts as an internal orthotic device that keeps the foot in the correct position while the medial soft tissues are healing. The authors think also that some degree of arthrofibrosis generates at the subtalar joint that prevents it from subluxating after implant removal. In our experience, the incidence of implant intolerance with sinus tarsi pain is very frequent. When the authors recommend a subtalar arthroereisis sinus tarsi implant to treat a stage IIA PTT dysfunction, the patient is informed about the possibility of postoperative sinus tarsi pain that may require a second surgery for implant removal.

SUMMARY

Subtalar arthroereisis, often combined with Achilles tendon lengthening, is a simple and effective way to treat flexible flatfoot in adults. The most common complication is pain in sinus tarsi, which usually disappears after removal of the implant. Midterm results are good and it does not hinder other treatments in the future.

REFERENCES

1. Noll KH. The use of orthotic devices in adult acquired flatfoot deformity. Foot Ankle Clin North Am 2001;6:25–36.
2. Chambers EF. An operation for the correction of flexible flat feet of adolescents. West J Surg Obstet Gynecol 1946;54:603–4.
3. Grice DS. An extra-articular arthrodesis of the subastragalar joint for correction of paralytic flat feet in Children. J Bone Joint Surg Am 1952;34:927–40.
4. Haraldsson S. Operative treatment of pes planovalgus staticus juvenilis. Acta Orthop Scand 1962;32:492–8.
5. Lelievre J. The valgus foot: current concepts and correction. Clin Orthop 1970;70: 43–55.
6. Viladot R, Pons M, Álvarez F, et al. Subtalar arthroereisis for posterior tibial tendon dysfunction: a preliminary report. Foot Ankle Int 2003;24:600–6.
7. Zaret DI, Myerson MS. Arthroereisis of the subtalar joint. Foot Ankle Clin North Am 2003;8:605–17.
8. Needleman RL. Current topic review: subtalar arthroereisis for correction of flexible flatfoot. Foot Ankle Int 2005;26:336–46.
9. Subotnick S. The subtalar joint lateral extra-articular arthroereisis: a follow-up report. J Am Podiatry Assoc 1977;32:27–33.
10. Smith SD, Millar EA. Arthroereisis by means of the subtalar polyethylene peg implant for correction of hindfoot pronation in children. Clin Orthop 1983;181:15–25.
11. Viladot A. Surgical treatment of the child's flatfoot. Clin Orthop 1992;283:34–8.
12. Vogler H. Subtalar joint blocking operations for pathological pronation syndromes. In: McGlamery ED, editor. Comprehensive textbook of foot surgery. Baltimore: William & Wilkins; 1987. p. 466–82.
13. Johnson KA, Strom DE. Tibialis posterior tendon dysfunction. Clin Orthop 1989;239: 196–206.

14. Myerson MS. Adult acquired flatfoot deformity. J Bone Joint Surg Am 1996;78:780–92.

15. Bluman E, Title CI, Myerson MS. Posterior tibial tendon rupture: a refined classification system. Foot Ankle Clin North Am 2007;12:233–49.

16. Hill K, Saar WE, Lee TH, et al. Stage II flatfoot: what fails and why. Foot Ankle Clin North Am 2003;8:91–104.

17. Mann R, Thompson FM. Rupture of the posterior tibial tendon causing flat foot: surgical treatment. J Bone Joint Surg 1985;67:556–61.

18. Kitaoka HB, Luo ZP, An KN. Reconstructive operations for acquired flatfoot: biomechanical evaluation. Foot Ankle Int 1998;19:303–4.

19. Gazdag AR, Cracchiolo A. Rupture of the posterior tibial tendon. Evaluation of injury of the spring ligament and clinical assessment of tendon transfer and ligament repair. J Bone Joint Surg 1997;79A:675–81.

20. Arangio GA, Reinert KL, Salathe EP. A biomechanical model of the effect of subtalar arthroereisis on the adult flexible flat foot. Clin Biomech 2004;19:847–52.

21. Saxena A, Nguyen A. Preliminary radiographic findings and sizing implications on patients undergoing bioabsorbable subtalar arthroereisis. J Foot Ankle Surg 2007;46:175–80.

22. Vedantam R, Capelli AM, Schoenecker PL. Subtalar arthroereisis for the correction of planovalgus foot in children with neuromuscular disorders. J Pediatr Orthop 1998;18:294–8.

23. Rocket AK, Mangum G, Mendicino SS. Bilateral intraosseous cystic formation in the talus: a complication of subtalar arthroereisis. J Foot Ankle Surg 1996;37:421–5.

24. Siff TE, Granberry WM. Avascular necrosis of the talus following subtalar arthroereisis with a polyethylene endoprosthesis: a case report. Foot Ankle Int 2000;21:247–9.

25. Kuwada GT, Dockery GL. Complications following traumatic incidents with STA-peg procedures. J Foot Surg 1988;27:236–9.

26. Dalton GP, Wapner KL, Hecht PJ. Complications of Achilles and posterior tibial tendon surgeries. Clin Orthop 2001;391:133–9.

27. Giannini S. Operative treatment of the flatfoot: why and how. Foot Ankle Int 1998;19: 52–8.

28. Maxwell JR, Carro A, Sun C. Use of the Maxwell-Brancheau arthroereisis implant for the correction of posterior tibial tendon dysfunction. Clin Podiatr Med Surg 1999;16: 479–89.

29. Needleman RL. A surgical approach for flexible flatfeet in adults including a subtalar arthroereisis with the MBA sinus tarsi implant. Foot Int 2006;27:9–18.

30. Adelman VR, Szczepanski JA, Adelman RP. Radiographic evaluation of endoscopic gastrocnemius recession, subtalar joint arthroereisis, and flexor tendon transfer for surgical correction of stage II posterior tibial tendon dysfunction: a pilot study. J Foot Ankle Surg 2008;47:400–8.

31. Giannini S, Ceccarelli F, Vannini F, et al. Operative treatment of flatfoot with talocalcaneal coalition. Clin Orthop 2003;411:178–87.

32. Myerson MS, Badekas A, Schon LC. Treatment of stage II posterior tibial tendon deficiency with flexor digitorum tendon transfer and calcaneal osteotomy. Foot Ankle Int 2004;25:445–50.

33. Greene DL, Thompson MC, Gesink DS. Anatomic study of the medial neurovascular structures in relation to calcaneal osteotomy. Foot Ankle Int 2001;22:569–71.

34. Schon LC. Subtalar arthroereisis: a new exploration of an old concept. Foot Ankle Clin North Am 2007;12:329–39, vii.

35. Bruyn JM, Cerniglia MW, Chaney DM. Combination of Evans calcaneal osteotomy and STA-peg arthroereisis for correction of severe pes valgo planus deformity. J Foot Ankle Surg 1999;38:339–46.

Medial Column Procedures in the Correction of Adult Acquired Flatfoot Deformity

Jeremy J. McCormick, MD*, Jeffrey E. Johnson, MD

KEYWORDS

- Adult acquired flatfoot defomity • Cotton osteotomy • Forefoot varus
- Medial column osteoarthritis

KEY POINTS

- Forefoot varus is a common finding associated with the adult acquired flatfoot deformity (AFFD).
- Physical examination of the foot, when the hindfoot has been corrected to neutral, is the best method to determine if forefoot varus exists and whether surgical correction is needed.
- Forefoot varus owing to mild instability of the naviculocuneiform joint or the first tarsometatarsal joint is treated with a plantarflexion opening wedge osteotomy (Cotton osteotomy) of the first cuneiform.
- Forefoot varus owing to medial column osteoarthritis or significant instability is treated with arthrodesis of the involved joint(s) to restore the "tripod" of the foot.

Adult acquired flatfoot deformity (AAFD) is a global term that applies to patients with varying degrees of hindfoot valgus, forefoot abduction, and forefoot varus. Most commonly, a patient complains of medial hindfoot pain and swelling with a variable degree of progressive pes planovalgus. The most common cause of AAFD is posterior tibial tendon (PTT) dysfunction.[1] Function of the PTT is critical because it contributes to the static stability of the foot along with the spring ligament complex.[2] Failure of the PTT to maintain the arch of the foot can lead to progressive hindfoot valgus and collapse of the medial column through the first metatarsocuneiform joint (also known as the first tarsometatarsal [TMT] joint), the naviculocuneiform (NC) joint, and/or the talonavicular (TN) joint.[2] Other etiologies of AAFD include pathology such as post-traumatic deformity, osteoarthritis, inflammatory arthritis, Charcot neuroarthropathy, and neuromuscular disorders.[3,4] Numerous combinations of bone and soft-tissue

Department of Orthopedic Surgery, Foot and Ankle Service, Washington University School of Medicine, 660 South Euclid Avenue, St Louis, MO 63110, USA
* Corresponding author.
E-mail address: mccormickj@wudosis.wustl.edu

Foot Ankle Clin N Am 17 (2012) 283–298
http://dx.doi.org/10.1016/j.fcl.2012.03.003
1083-7515/12/$ – see front matter © 2012 Published by Elsevier Inc.

procedures have been described to address the different types of pes planovalgus deformity without a clear consensus on a treatment algorithm.[2,5–15]

BACKGROUND

The typical history given by a patient with an acquired flatfoot deformity secondary to PTT insufficiency is a progressive change in the shape of their foot over time. The patient describes increasing pain and difficulty with weight-bearing activities. Typically, there is no specific instance where the foot changed form, or "collapsed."

Physical examination begins with an observation of the standing alignment of the foot and ankle to evaluate the extent of hindfoot valgus, midfoot pronation, and forefoot abduction. Assessment of neurovascular and motor function is performed to rule out other causes of tendon dysfunction and ensure that the remaining muscle function in normal. The PTT is examined with the patient seated by asking them to invert the foot while maintaining a plantarflexed and everted posture to the foot so as to reduce inversion by the anterior tibial tendon that may mask PTT weakness. This maneuver typically demonstrates weakness of the PTT compared with the contralateral side.

In the early stages of disease, deformity of the foot remains flexible and correctible; however, in later stages the deformity remains fixed. The best way to evaluate the ability to correct a foot deformity to a more normal posture is on seated examination. Hindfoot valgus is typically corrected through the subtalar joint by grasping the calcaneus with one hand and internally rotating the calcaneus while stabilizing the ankle and talus with the other hand. If the hindfoot can be corrected to a normal posture through the subtalar joint and the midfoot can be corrected through the transverse tarsal joint, then it is felt to be a correctible deformity. At this time, while holding the hindfoot in neutral, any gastrocnemius or soleus contracture can be assessed with the use of the Silfverskiöld test.

Persistent hindfoot valgus and collapse of the medial column eventually results in forefoot varus, which may be exhibited by significant first ray elevation or global forefoot varus at the transverse tarsal joint.[16] Deformity through the medial column should be evaluated with the patient in the seated position. The hindfoot is placed in a "neutral position" by centering the navicular over the talar head.[17] The deformity is confirmed by palpating the medial border of the foot and the relationship of the navicular tuberosity to the talar head. As the hindfoot is held in this position with one hand, the opposite hand is used to passively bring the ankle to neutral dorsiflexion by placing force on the plantar aspect of the fourth and fifth metatarsal heads. At this point, the relationship of the first and fifth metatarsals is evaluated by viewing the foot "head-on" to determine the degree of elevation of the first ray relative to the fifth ray which is known as the degree of forefoot varus (**Fig. 1**).[18]

Stability of the first ray is assessed with the patient in a seated position by stabilizing the lesser four metatarsals with one hand and then using the opposite hand to manipulate the first metatarsal. The dorsiflexion and plantarflexion of the first ray in relation to the rest of the foot is assessed to determine if there is excessive motion or if there is pain or crepitus with range of motion.

In addition to the physical examination, radiographs play an important role in determining the etiology of AAFD as well as assessing the deformity of a patient's foot. Weight-bearing radiographs of the foot and ankle should be obtained for proper evaluation. On a normal weight-bearing anteroposterior and lateral radiograph, the calcaneocuboid joint should be at the same level as the TN joint. With AAFD, the foot radiographs show the appearance of a short lateral column compared with the medial

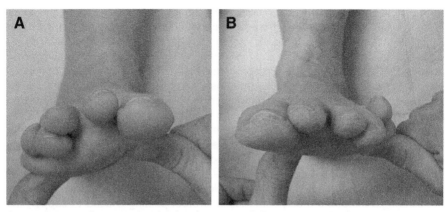

Fig. 1. Photograph comparing (A) forefoot varus deformity with the first metatarsal head elevated above the fifth metatarsal head in the coronal plane and (B) normal forefoot alignment.

column, with the TN joint approximately 3 to 5 mm distal to the calcaneocuboid joint.[19] Additionally, the anteroposterior radiograph helps to quantify forefoot abduction through evaluation of the TN coverage angle. This is measured by determining the amount of the talar head that is "covered" by the navicular, with a smaller degree of coverage corresponding with increased forefoot abduction.

On the weight-bearing lateral radiograph, the medial column of the foot can be carefully evaluated. The lateral talo–first metatarsal angle, also known as Meary's angle, is measured between the line drawn representing the longitudinal axis of the talus and that of the first metatarsal. Normal is considered measurements from +5 to −5 degrees. Measurements less than −5 degrees are considered to have pes planus. Another angular measurement that can be measured on a weight-bearing lateral radiograph is the calcaneal pitch. This is the angle formed by the intersection of a line drawn along the plantar surface of the calcaneus and a line drawn parallel to the ground. Normal measurement for calcaneal pitch is 10–30°, thus less than 10° would be considered abnormally flat (**Fig. 2**).

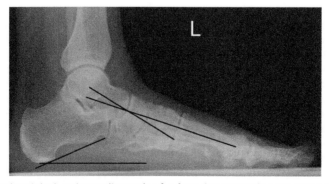

Fig. 2. Lateral weight-bearing radiograph of a foot demonstrating Meary's angle (normal +5° to −5°) and calcaneal pitch angle (normal, 10° to 30°).

In addition to angular measurements, the joints of the medial column should be carefully evaluated on the weight-bearing lateral radiograph. Instability at the TMT, NC, or TN joints may result in asymmetry at the joint where there may be a relative plantar gap at the joint space or subluxation. Further, the medial column joints may show evidence of degenerative change such as joint space narrowing, subchondral sclerosis, or osteophytes. Identifying the unstable or arthritic joint along the medial column is important because this information will help guide the surgical treatment plan if nonoperative modalities fail.

Nonoperative treatment for medial column deformity or instability with a foot orthosis may be helpful, especially if the patient has a flexible or correctible deformity as characterized on physical examination. A custom-molded, semi-rigid foot orthosis for arch support is posted at the medial heel and the lateral forefoot to help correct foot pronation and forefoot varus. If the forefoot varus is rigid, then an accommodative, semi-rigid molded orthosis with medial forefoot posting is used to support the forefoot in the varus posture. If these options are unsuccessful, or if the patient has a more rigid deformity that is not easily corrected with an orthosis, the patient can use a custom molded brace such as a plastic and leather composite lace up brace (ie, an Arizona brace) or a rigid ankle–foot–orthosis with a molded foot orthosis inside the brace.

For AAFD, there are numerous surgical options that include tendon repair, tendon transfer, osteotomies, fusions, and combinations of these procedures.[2,5–14] The operative procedures chosen must address the etiology of the AAFD and, most important, must address all the components of the deformity. If the deformity is flexible or passively correctible on physical examination and not associated with degenerative joint disease, then a reconstructive option utilizing osteotomies can be considered. If the deformity is rigid or not passively correctible, then one must employ a triple arthrodesis (fusion of the subtalar, TN, and calcaneocuboid joints) to correct the deformity appropriately.

With flexible deformity, most commonly PTT dysfunction, the reconstructive procedure includes a medial soft tissue reconstruction that involves a flexor digitorum longus tendon transfer to the navicular to augment or replace the PTT in addition to repair or imbrication of the spring ligament if needed. Additionally, the gastrocnemius and soleus complex is addressed with lengthening as needed to decrease the hindfoot valgus force and resultant influence on the forefoot deformity.[20,21] Reconstruction or repair of the medial soft tissue structures helps to restore function to the foot; however, the underlying flatfoot deformity would eventually result in attenuation and failure of the repair.[22] As such, it is important to correct any underlying deformity with bony procedures.

Options for bony correction commonly include a medial displacement calcaneal osteotomy to primarily correct the hindfoot valgus deformity or a lateral column lengthening to correct forefoot abduction. However, these procedures do not address the forefoot varus component of the AAFD.[23] Even a triple arthrodesis may not completely correct forefoot varus if the deformity is distal to the TN joint. Without appropriate correction of the flatfoot deformity, the patient retains some level of deformity and has altered biomechanics with excessive weight-bearing on the lateral border of the foot and possible overload of the deltoid ligament of the ankle.

Numerous options exist for correction of forefoot varus through the medial column.[16] The appropriate choice is based on proper identification of the location of deformity and identification of abnormal or arthritic joints. The focus of this article is on two such medial column procedures: the Cotton osteotomy (plantarflexion opening wedge medial cuneiform osteotomy) and the first TMT fusion.

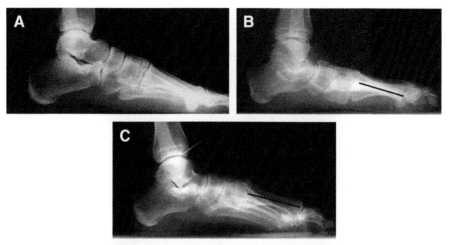

Fig. 3. Lateral weight-bearing radiographs demonstrating (A) normal forefoot posture, (B) the contralateral foot of the same patient with AAFD whose lateral radiograph is taken in a weight-bearing stance with hindfoot valgus, and (C) the same patient with AAFD whose lateral radiograph was taken with the hindfoot repositioned into neutral. Note the forefoot varus, which becomes quite evident as the heel is positioned in neutral, thereby elevating the medial column. The first metatarsal head is now elevated and the fifth metatarsal head is now able to be visualized on the lateral radiograph.

THE COTTON MEDIAL CUNEIFORM OSTEOTOMY

In 1936, Cotton[5] described a procedure to assist in correction of the flatfoot deformity that used an opening wedge medial cuneiform osteotomy to plantarflex the first ray. With this procedure, he theorized that the "triangle of support" would be restored to the foot and allow the patient to have improved function by restoring the mechanics of weight-bearing.[5] Since Cotton's original report, little has been written on the use of this medial cuneiform osteotomy as part of flatfoot deformity correction.[5,10]

Indications

A plantarflexion opening wedge medial cuneiform osteotomy should be used as an adjunct to reconstruction of a flatfoot deformity. Primarily it is used to correct forefoot varus with elevation of the medial column where the deformity is located at the first TMT joint or the NC joint.[17] This forefoot varus is typically identified preoperatively on physical examination and is further evaluated with preoperative weight-bearing radiographs (see **Fig. 1**; **Fig. 3**).

The Cotton osteotomy is a joint-sparing procedure; thus, the first TMT joint should be stable or have only mild instability on physical examination. Further, there should not be any radiographic evidence of joint abnormality such as plantar gapping on the lateral weight-bearing radiograph or findings of significant osteoarthritis. If the lateral x-ray demonstrates marked dorsal subluxation of the first metatarsal in relation to the medial cuneiform or if there are findings of arthritis, cuneiform osteotomy is contra-indicated.[17] In these cases, arthrodesis of the first TMT joint is indicated. Further contraindications to the Cotton osteotomy include deformity that is greater than what a 5- to 8-mm plantarflexion bone block can correct.[17] In these situations, more proximal procedures such as reduction and fusion of the NC or TN joints are

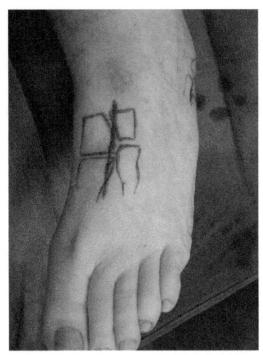

Fig. 4. A dorsal longitudinal incision is used that is centered over the medial cuneiform. Care is taken to stay medial to the dorsalis pedis artery and deep peroneal nerve.

indicated. Additionally, a fixed forefoot deformity through the transverse tarsal joints should be addressed with correction at this more proximal level rather than through a cuneiform osteotomy.

Most commonly, the Cotton osteotomy is performed as a last step in surgical reconstruction of the AAFD. Typically, the other hindfoot osteotomies would have been completed and fixed in their corrected position. After the medial soft-tissue repair and tendon transfers are prepared for fixation, the static posture of the newly corrected foot is evaluated. The amount of residual forefoot varus is assessed both clinically and with a lateral intraoperative x-ray; and if significant deformity remains, it should be corrected to restore the "triangle of support."[4]

Technique

The patient is positioned supine on the operating room table for the flatfoot reconstruction procedure. A bump is placed under the ipsilateral buttock to internally rotate the affected leg and a tourniquet is placed around the thigh. If the surgeon elects to use an autograft, the donor iliac crest is prepped and draped along with the operative leg. Under tourniquet, a dorsal longitudinal incision is made over the level of the medial cuneiform joint (**Fig. 4**). The skin and subcutaneous tissues are carefully dissected down to the level of the extensor hallucis longus (EHL) and extensor hallucis brevis (EHB) tendons. The EHL is retracted medially and the EHB is retracted laterally. Care is taken to be sure the dorsalis pedis artery and deep peroneal nerve are lateral to the field of work. The dorsal portion of the medial cuneiform is exposed.

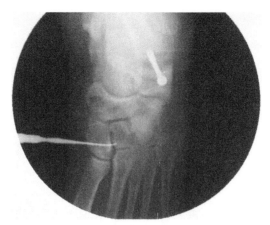

Fig. 5. A metallic instrument is used to identify the proposed location of the transverse osteotomy of the medial cuneiform.

At this point, the C-arm fluoroscopy is used to identify the mid-portion of the cuneiform. It is at this level that the osteotomy is performed (**Fig. 5**). A microsagittal saw is then used to create a transverse osteotomy from dorsal to plantar through the midportion of the medial cuneiform (**Fig. 6**). On lateral C-arm images, this tends to be at or just proximal to the level of the second TMT joint. The saw is used to cut the bone up to, but not through, the plantar cortex of the cuneiform. An osteotome is then used to propagate the cuneiform osteotomy in a greenstick manner. It is important to leave the plantar periosteum and ligamentous attachments intact so that the osteotomy does not risk displacement or distraction. That same osteotome is then pulled distally and used as a lever to plantarflex the first ray through the newly created osteotomy (**Fig. 7**). The foot is then evaluated both clinically and with lateral C-arm imaging to determine the amount of correction that is needed to restore Cotton's "triangle of support" and the width of the osteotomy gap is measured. Generally, a 5- to 8-mm wedge of bone is needed to plantarflex the first metatarsal so that clinically and radiographically it rests in line with the fifth metatarsal head.

The graft is obtained next. A tricortical iliac crest wedge has been described, although many types of bone grafts may suffice, and it is surgeon's preference whether to employ autograft or allograft. The graft is cut into a triangular wedge with a microsagittal saw to the appropriate size, so that the graft's cancellous surfaces opposes the cancellous surfaces of the native cuneiform. The cortical surfaces of the graft should rest dorsally, medially, and laterally. A narrow osteotome is then used to lever open the graft site and the graft is gently impacted in place with a bone tamp. Fixation of the graft is the surgeon's preference and may include a K-wire, a single cannulated screw, a compression staple, or a small plate (**Fig. 8**). The author's preference is a single, 0.062-inch smooth K-wire for percutaneous fixation across the osteotomy, which is removed at 4 to 6 weeks. Some surgeons use no internal fixation. Recently, a wedge plate as well as a metallic wedge have been developed and marketed; however, we have no experience using these devices.[24] The wounds are closed and the patient is splinted. The postoperative protocol may depend on the other concomitant procedures performed at the time of the Cotton osteotomy. Typically, the patient remains non–weight-bearing and casted for a total of 6 weeks from the time of surgery. At that point, assuming the radiographs show signs of

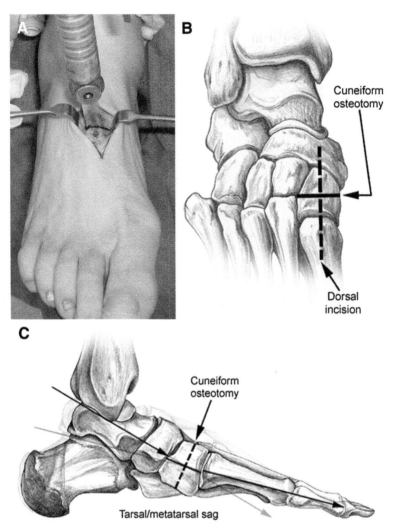

Fig. 6. (*A*) A transverse osteotomy is made through the midportion of the cuneiform using a microsagittal saw. (*B*) Drawing demonstrating the typical location of the cuneiform osteotomy at or just proximal to the level of the second tarsometatarsal joint. (*C*) Drawing demonstrating the location of the cuneiform osteotomy. Osteotomy is made perpendicular to the long access of the bone.

healing and the patient has no significant tenderness, the patient is allowed to bear weight in a protective boot. With standard progression, they begin weaning from the boot at about 10 weeks after surgery (**Fig. 9**).

Results

In his original article, Cotton stated that "the operation is simple, not painful, and . . . in the short series of cases done since I devised this operation, there has been no trouble in any."[5] More recent literature has supported this claim and shown the procedure to be straightforward and predictable, with minimal morbidity. In one

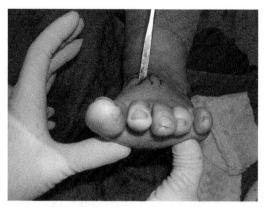

Fig. 7. An osteotome is inserted into the cuneiform osteotomy and used to lever the first ray into plantarflexion, correcting forefoot varus. The first metatarsal head is corrected until it comes in line with the fifth metatarsal head in the coronal plane.

clinical review of the Cotton procedure, Hirose and Johnson reviewed a series of 16 patients who underwent correction of their residual forefoot varus with a plantarflexion medial cuneiform osteotomy.[17] They utilized iliac crest autograft and internal fixation and found no incidence of nonunion or malunion. At the time of follow-up, all patients had mild to no pain with ambulation. Further, comparison of preoperative to postoperative weight-bearing radiographs showed an average improvement in Meary's angle of 14° (−13° preoperative, 1° postoperative), demonstrating significant correction of forefoot varus.[17]

In another recent clinical series, Lutz and Myerson[25] reported on 101 medial cuneiform osteotomies performed in conjunction with a comprehensive flatfoot reconstructive procedure. This series did not report any nonunions, supporting the thought that the Cotton osteotomy heals predictably. Further, they demonstrated a statistically significant rate of improvement in Meary's angle from a preoperative average value of −23° to an average postoperative value of −1°.

Biomechanically, research has examined the weight-bearing characteristics of feet before and after Cotton osteotomy. Scott and colleageus[26] used cadaveric specimens to evaluate plantar pressures and loading characteristics after a medial displacement calcaneal osteotomy, lateral column lengthening, and Cotton osteotomy.[26] They found that the plantarflexion medial cuneiform osteotomy did increase average plantar pressure within the medial forefoot, but did not create off-loading of the lateral forefoot where the plantar pressures remained similar before and after the Cotton osteotomy. Benthien and associates[27] found conflicting results in a similar cadaveric study by showing that the lateral forefoot pressure decreased with the addition of a medial cuneiform osteotomy.

There have been some complications found with the use of this procedure. In Hirose and Johnson's series, 1 patient had a symptomatic screw that was removed, but there were no problems with nonunion or residual pain.[17] In Lutz and Myerson's larger series,[25] there were 10 postoperative complications attributed at least in part to the Cotton osteotomy: 3 symptomatic screws, 2 bony exostosis, 1 sesamoid pain, 1 plantar fasciitis, 2 lateral column overload symptoms, and 1 recurrence of flatfoot deformity. Overall, the Cotton osteotomy has proven straightforward and useful in correcting residual forefoot varus in AAFD and should be carefully considered when

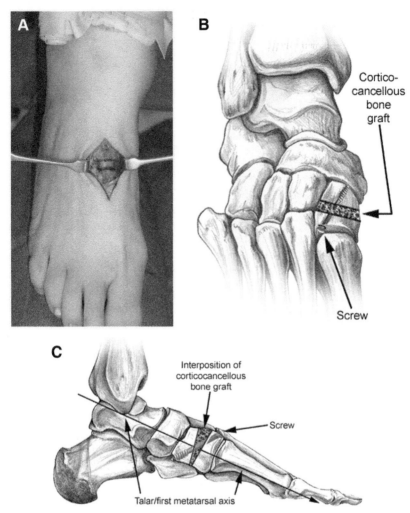

Fig. 8. (A) Intraoperative photograph of the medial cuneiform osteotomy with graft in place. (B) Diagram of the foot from a dorsal view demonstrating the location of the interposition graft with screw fixation. (C) Diagram of the lateral foot demonstrating the insertion of the interposition bone graft with an oblique partially threaded screw for fixation.

there is no abnormality at the first TMT joint. Further, it allows for preservation of the first TMT joint and NC joint, permitting normal motion through the foot after reconstruction of Cotton's "triangle of support."

TMT JOINT FUSION

In 1934, Lapidus[28] described a procedure for use in correction of hallux valgus where a distal soft-tissue procedure and medial eminence resection was performed along with arthrodesis of the first and second TMT joints. Since then, it has evolved to include arthrodesis of only the first TMT joint.[29] Although its original intent was for use in correcting hallux valgus, surgeons have expanded the indications of the first TMT arthrodesis by using it to correct medial column deformity in AAFD.[20]

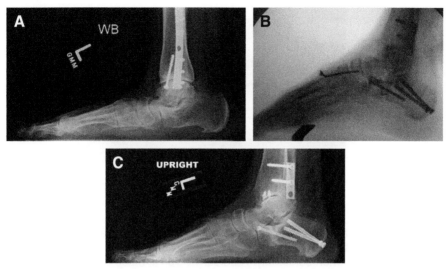

Fig. 9. (*A*) Preoperative lateral weight-bearing radiograph of a foot with AAFD. (*B*) Immediate postoperative C-arm image after surgical correction. The patient has undergone a medial displacement calcaneal osteotomy, a lateral column lengthening with interposition graft, a medial soft tissue reconstruction with flexor digitorum longus transfer to the navicular, and a Cotton osteotomy—fixed with a single, 0.062-inch K-wire. (*C*) Lateral weight-bearing radiograph after reconstruction has healed and patient is ambulatory.

Indications

Much like the Cotton osteotomy, the first TMT arthrodesis should be used as an adjunct to a comprehensive flatfoot reconstruction. It is used to correct residual forefoot varus in the AAFD when the deformity is identified to be primarily through the first TMT joint. As with the Cotton osteotomy, indications for this procedure are determined after careful preoperative physical examination and evaluation of preoperative weight-bearing radiographs. The first TMT arthrodesis should be employed when forefoot varus remains after correction of the hindfoot and there is clinical or radiographic evidence of significant joint arthrosis or instability. On physical examination, this is identified as gross instability or hypermobility of the first TMT joint or pain and crepitus with range of motion of the joint. Radiographically, abnormality of the first TMT joint is seen as asymmetric plantar gapping on weight-bearing lateral view, joint malalignment, or subluxation on weight-bearing lateral view (**Fig. 10**), or evidence of arthritic changes at the first TMT joint, such as joint space narrowing or sclerosis. With these findings, a joint-sparing procedure such as the Cotton osteotomy is no longer a predictable option because of the concern for residual joint instability or pain. As with the Cotton osteotomy, however, it is important to assess whether a first TMT fusion will correct the deformity sufficiently or whether a more proximal procedure such as a NC or TN fusion is necessary.

The first TMT fusion is typically performed as a last step in the reconstruction of the AAFD. After the hindfoot correction has been completed, the posture of the foot should be evaluated both clinically and radiographically. If significant forefoot varus deformity remains and there is gross instability, hypermobility, or degenerative change at the first TMT joint, then a first TMT fusion can be used to correct the deformity.

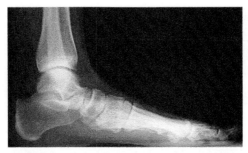

Fig. 10. Weight-bearing lateral radiograph demonstrating instability at the first TMT joint.

Technique

The patient is positioned supine, with a bump under the ipsilateral buttock and a tourniquet around the thigh. The leg is prepped and draped in exactly the same manner as for the Cotton osteotomy. A dorsal incision is made over the level of the first TMT joint and the skin and subcutaneous tissues are carefully dissected until the EHL and EHB tendons are visualized and retracted medially and laterally, respectively. Care is taken to ensure the dorsalis pedis artery and deep peroneal nerve remain lateral to the surgical site, and, if they are visualized, they are retracted laterally with the EHB tendon. At this point, the first TMT joint is identified and a longitudinal incision is made through the joint capsule, which is then elevated medially and laterally to expose the joint. If there is any concern about identification of the first TMT joint, a C-arm fluoroscopy unit can be used for verification.

Once the joint is identified and exposed, the joint surfaces are prepared by removing all of the cartilage from the proximal aspect of the first metatarsal and the distal aspect of the medial cuneiform. This is completed with the use of instruments such as osteotomes, curettes, and rongeurs. It should be noted that the first TMT joint is quite deep from dorsal to plantar, measuring on the order of 3 cm. As such, care should be taken to prepare the full extent of the joint and avoid dorsiflexion through the arthrodesis, which would be created by incomplete preparation of the most plantar aspect of the joint. A lamina spreader or distraction apparatus using pins in the bone is helpful to gain access to the entire first TMT joint. Once all of the cartilage has been removed, the subchondral joint surface is further prepared by drilling or petaling the bone to increase the bleeding surface area for fusion.

After the surfaces are prepared, the first TMT joint must be reduced to the appropriate position of fusion. Clinical examination and C-arm fluoroscopy images are used to ensure that the medial column is being appropriately plantarflexed to correct the forefoot varus. As described for the Cotton osteotomy, this is accomplished by ensuring that the first metatarsal head rests in line with the fifth metatarsal head clinically and radiographically. If anatomic reduction of the first TMT joint does not correct the forefoot varus, resection of a small plantar wedge from the metatarsal base or the use of an interposition wedge graft much like a Cotton osteotomy may augment the correction. As with the plantarflexion cuneiform osteotomy, if a tricortical iliac crest autograft or allograft is used, the joint surfaces are flattened with a microsagittal saw and a wedge is cut to the size that creates the appropriate amount of plantarflexion through the first TMT fusion site. An osteotome is used to lever open the joint into an improved, plantarflexed posture and the graft is gently impacted into place. As an alternative to an opening wedge graft, one might consider a plantar

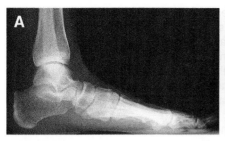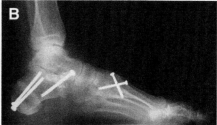

Fig. 11. (*A*) Preoperative lateral weight-bearing radiograph of a patient with AAFD and first TMT instability. (*B*) Lateral weight-bearing radiograph of a patient after reconstruction has healed. The patient has undergone a medial displacement calcaneal osteotomy, a lateral column lengthening with interposition graft, a medial soft tissue reconstruction with flexor digitorum longus transfer to the navicular, and a first TMT joint arthrodesis—fixed with crossed lag screws.

closing wedge osteotomy at the level of the first TMT joint. The authors have minimal experience with plantar closing wedge osteotomy of the cuneiform for the correction of forefoot varus and have been able to correct the majority of medial column deformities with a 5- to 8-mm dorsal bone wedge. However, for a more severe dorsiflexion deformity of the medial column with a normal first TMT and TN joint, we would favor either a double bone block opening wedge osteotomy as has been described for a dorsal bunion correction[30] or a correction and stabilization through the naviculo-first cuneiform joint as similar to the Miller flatfoot procedure, the modified Hoke–Miller or the Durham plasty procedures.[7,9,31]

Fixation for the first TMT fusion is most commonly dual compression crossed screws or a single compression screw with a dorsal plate. The soft tissues and incision are then carefully closed and the patient is splinted. The postoperative protocol varies based on concomitant procedures that have been performed; however, typically the patient is casted and non–weight-bearing for 6 weeks from the time of their operation. At that point, they are typically transitioned to a boot for progressive weight bearing, assuming that the clinical and radiographic examinations do not raise concern for delayed healing. At 10 to 12 weeks after their surgery, the patient is usually transitioning from their boot to a shoe and progressing with activities as clinically tolerated (**Fig. 11**).

Results

In the past, there has been apprehension about performing the first TMT arthrodesis because of concerns for rates of nonunion. Some authors have cited rates as high as 12%; however, a recent paper by Thompson and colleagues[32] had a better union rate. In their review of 182 patients who had undergone fusion of the first TMT joint for correction of hallux valgus or as a component to reconstruction of AAFD, the nonunion rate was only 4%. Of those, only half were symptomatic and required revision surgery. Further analysis shows that, of those patients who underwent first TMT fusion as part of a flatfoot reconstruction, there were no instances of nonunion. They attributed their low rate of nonunion to careful bone preparation, addition of bone graft, and the use of Achilles or gastrocnemius lengthening procedures as indicated to unload stresses through the forefoot.

Cadaveric biomechanical studies have investigated various constructs for Lapidus arthrodesis. One study showed no significant difference between locked plate fixation and dual crossed lag screw fixation in terms of rigidity.[33] Two studies, however, showed greater rigidity at first TMT fusion site with a locked plate as compared with dual crossed lag screws.[34,35] DeVries and associates[36] compared the clinical outcome of these fixation methods and found a significant increase in union rate when a locked plate was used as compared with the dual crossed screw technique. The dual screw technique did have an acceptable union rate of almost 90%, however, suggesting it to be a viable option. In our practice, we customarily use a lag screw and dorsal locked plate.

Although Thompson and colleagues[32] showed a high rate of union that may not be attainable by all surgeons, at the least it suggests that the procedure is safe and reasonable. Outside of the cited nonunions, there were 6 superficial wound infections treated with oral antibiotics and 2 local wound breakdowns requiring wound care in addition to antibiotic treatment. No deep infections or incidence of more severe complications were identified. The procedure does sacrifice mobility of the first TMT joint; however, in the face of first TMT hypermobility or arthritic change at the first TMT joint, Lapidus fusion is a procedure that does quite well as an adjunct to a comprehensive flatfoot reconstruction.

SUMMARY

AAFD is a complex problem with a wide variety of treatment options. No single procedure or group of procedures can be applied to all patients with AAFD because of the variety of underlying etiology and grades of deformity. As the posture of the foot progresses into hindfoot valgus and forefoot abduction through attenuation of the medial structures of the foot, the medial column begins to change shape. The first ray elevates and the joints of the medial column may begin to collapse. Careful physical examination and review of weight-bearing radiographs determines which patients have an associated forefoot varus deformity that may require correction at the time of flatfoot reconstruction.

Correction of an AAFD requires a combination of soft-tissue procedures to restore dynamic inversion power and bony procedures to correct the hindfoot and midfoot malalignments. If after these corrections forefoot varus deformity remains, the surgeon should consider use of a medial column procedure to recreate the "triangle of support" of the foot that Cotton described.[5] If the elevation of the medial column is identified to be at the first NC or the first TMT joint, then the joint should be carefully examined for evidence of instability, hypermobility, or arthritic change. If none of these problems exist, then the surgeon can consider use of the joint-sparing Cotton medial cuneiform osteotomy to correct residual forefoot varus. However, if instability, hypermobility, or arthritic change is present, then the surgeon should consider use of an arthrodesis of the involved joint to correct residual forefoot varus. Either procedure provides a safe and predictable correction to the medial column as part of a comprehensive surgical correction of AAFD.

REFERENCES

1. Funk DA, Cass JR, Johnson KA. Acquired adult flat foot secondary to posterior tibial-tendon pathology. J Bone Joint Surg Am 1986;68:95–102.
2. Pedowitz WJ, Kovatis P. Flatfoot in the Adult. J Am Acad Orthop Surg 1995;3:293–302.
3. Mann DA. Acquired flat foot in adults. Clin Orthop 1983;181:46–51.
4. Myerson MS. Acquired flat foot deformity. J Bone Joint Surg Am 1996;78:780–92.
5. Cotton FJ. Foot statics and surgery. N Engl J Med 1936:353–62.

6. Duncan JW, Lovell WW. Modified Hoke-Miller flatfoot procedure. Clin Orthop Relat Res 1983:24–7.
7. Hoke M. An operation for the correction of extremely relaxed flat feet. J Bone Joint Surg 1931:773.
8. Johnson JE, Cohen BE, DiGiovanni BF, et al. Subtalar arthrodesis with flexor digitorum longus transfer and spring ligament repair for treatment of posterior tibial tendon insufficiency. Foot Ankle Int 2000;21:722–9.
9. Miller OL. A plastic flatfoot operation. J Bone Joint Surg 1927:84.
10. Mosca VS. Calcaneal lengthening for valgus deformity of the hindfoot. Results in children who had severe, symptomatic flatfoot and skewfoot. J Bone Joint Surg Am 1995;77:500–12.
11. Myerson MS, Corrigan J, Thompson F, et al. Tendon transfer combined with calcaneal osteotomy for treatment of posterior tibial tendon insufficiency: a radiological investigation. Foot Ankle Int 1995;16:712–8.
12. Sands A, Grujic L, Sangeorzan BJ, et al. Lateral column lengthening through the calcaneocubiod joint: an alternative to triple arthrodesis for correction of flatfoot. In: AOFAS Annual Meeting. Orlando (FL), 1995.
13. Toolan BC, Sangeorzan BJ, Hansen ST Jr. Complex reconstruction for the treatment of dorsolateral peritalar subluxation of the foot. Early results after distraction arthrodesis of the calcaneocuboid joint in conjunction with stabilization of, and transfer of the flexor digitorum longus tendon to, the midfoot to treat acquired pes planovalgus in adults. J Bone Joint Surg Am 1999;81:1545–60.
14. Hirose CB. The use of plantarflexion opening wedge medial cuneiform osteotomy for correction of fixed forefoot varus associated with flatfoot deformity. In: AOFAS 33rd Annual Meeting. New Orleans (LA), 2003.
15. Hiller L, Pinney SJ. Surgical treatment of acquired flatfoot deformity: what is the state of practice among academic foot and ankle surgeons in 2002? Foot Ankle Int 2003;24:701–5.
16. Cohen BE, Ogden F. Medial column procedures in the acquired flatfoot deformity. Foot Ankle Clin 2007;12:287–99.
17. Johnson JE. Plantarflexion opening wedge cuneiform-1 osteotomy for correction of fixed forefoot varus. Techniques in Foot and Ankle Surgery 2004;3:2–8.
18. Alexander IJ. The foot: examination and diagnosis. New York: Churchill Livingstone; 1990.
19. Stephens HM, Walling AK, Solmen JD, et al. Subtalar repositional arthrodesis for adult acquired flatfoot. Clin Orthop Relat Res 1999;365:69–73.
20. Habbu R HS, Anderson JG, Bohay DR. Operative correction of arch collapse with forefoot deformity: a retrospective analysis of outcomes. Foot Ankle Int 2011;32:764–73.
21. Coughlin MJ, Kaz A. Correlation of Harris mats, physical exam, pictures, and radiographic measurements in adult flatfoot deformity. Foot Ankle Int 2009;30:604–12.
22. Michelson J,Conti S, Jahss MH. Surviving analysis of tendon transfer surgery for posterior tibial tendon rupture Orthop Trans 1992;16:30–1.
23. Neufeld SK, Myerson MS. Complications of surgical treatments for adult flatfoot deformities. Foot Ankle Clin 2001;6:179-91.
24. League AC, Parks BG, Schon LC. Radiographic and pedobarographic comparison of femoral head allograft versus block plate with dorsal opening wedge medial cuneiform osteotomy: a biomechanical study. Foot Ankle Int 2008;29:922–6.
25. Lutz M, Myerson M. Radiographic analysis of an opening wedge osteotomy of the medial cuneiform. Foot Ankle Int 2011;32:278–87.

26. Scott AT, Hendry TM, Iaquinto JM, et al. Plantar pressure analysis in cadaver feet after bony procedures commonly used in the treatment of stage II posterior tibial tendon insufficiency. Foot Ankle Int 2007;28:1143–53.

27. Benthien RA, Parks BG, Guyton GP, et al. Lateral column calcaneal lengthening, flexor digitorum longus transfer, and opening wedge medial cuneiform osteotomy for flexible flatfoot: a biomechanical study. Foot Ankle Int 2007;28:70–7.

28. Lapidus PW. The operative correction of the metatarsus primus varus in hallux valgus. Surg Gynecol Obstet 1934;58:183–91.

29. Sangeorzan BJ, Hansen ST Jr. Modified Lapidus procedure for hallux valgus. Foot Ankle 1989;9:262–6.

30. Johnson JE, Thomson AB, Yu JR. Double bone-block arthrodesis for the correction of dorsal bunion deformity. Techniques in Foot and Ankle Surgery 2007;6:170–4.

31. Caldwell GD. Surgical correction of relaxed flatfoot by the Durham flatfoot plasty. Clin Orthop 1953;2:221–6.

32. Thompson IM, Bohay DR, Anderson JG. Fusion rate of first tarsometatarsal arthrodesis in the modified Lapidus procedure and flatfoot reconstruction. Foot Ankle Int 2005;26:698–703.

33. Gruber F, Sinkov VS, Bae SY, et al. Crossed screws versus dorsomedial locking plate with compression screw for first metatarsocuneiform arthrodesis: a cadaver study. Foot Ankle Int 2008;29:927–30.

34. Klos K, Gueorguiev B, Muckley T, et al. Stability of medial locking plate and compression screw versus two crossed screws for lapidus arthrodesis. Foot Ankle Int 2010;31:158–63.

35. Scranton PE, Coetzee JC, Carreira D. Arthrodesis of the first metatarsocuneiform joint: a comparative study of fixation methods. Foot Ankle Int 2009;30:341–5.

36. DeVries JG, Granata JD, Hyer CF. Fixation of first tarsometatarsal arthrodesis: a retrospective comparative cohort of two techniques. Foot Ankle Int 2011;32:158–62.

Management of the Recurrent Deformity in a Flexible Foot Following Failure of Tendon Transfer: Is Arthrodesis Necessary?

Safet O. Hatic II, DO[a], Terrence M. Philbin, DO[b,c,*]

KEYWORDS

• Flexible flatfoot • Hindfoot arthrodesis • Posterior tibial tendon dysfunction

KEY POINTS

• Management of recurrent deformity in the flexible foot begins with a detailed history and physical examination, including review of previous operative records and, in some cases, evaluation of advanced imaging studies.

• The goals of treatment in the flexible flatfoot should include restoration of alignment and alleviation of pain while minimizing stiffness, maintaining motion, and avoiding overcorrection.

• Failure of soft tissue procedures and extra-articular corrections may necessitate limited hindfoot arthrodesis to facilitate maintenance of deformity correction.

• Particularly in younger, more high-demand patients, every effort must be made to preserve normal joint mechanics while alleviating pain and restoring functional alignment.

Johnson and Strom,[1] as well as other authors,[2–4] described a classification system for adult-acquired flatfoot deformity, which was later modified by Myerson and colleagues.[5] The classification is helpful as it relates to directing treatment. Broadly speaking, stages I and II represent flexible flatfoot deformities, while stages III and IV represent more severe fixed deformities. Most authors agree, in stage I flatfoot refractory to conservative nonoperative management and mild to moderate stage II

The authors have nothing to disclose.
[a] Orthopedic Associates of SW Ohio, 4160 Little York Road, Suite 10, Dayton, OH 45414, USA;
[b] Orthopedic Foot and Ankle Center, 300 Polaris Parkway, Suite 2000, Westerville, OH 43082, USA; [c] Foot and Ankle Service, Doctors Hospital Residency, Columbus, OH, USA
* Corresponding author. Orthopedic Foot and Ankle Center, 300 Polaris Parkway, Suite 2000, Westerville, OH 43082.
E-mail address: ofacresearch@orthofootankle.com

Foot Ankle Clin N Am 17 (2012) 299–307
http://dx.doi.org/10.1016/j.fcl.2012.03.007
1083-7515/12/$ – see front matter © 2012 Elsevier Inc. All rights reserved.

deformities, soft tissue reconstruction with posterior tibial tendon (PTT) debridement, tendon transfer, and medial displacement calcaneal osteotomy provide sufficient deformity correction while maintaining motion.[2,4–8] More severe stage II deformities represent a slightly more controversial treatment dilemma as some surgeons advocate lateral column lengthening with or without a calcaneal osteotomy, spring ligament repair, and/or primary limited arthrodesis procedures to achieve deformity correction.[6,9–12]

The goals of flatfoot treatment should include correction of deformity and alleviation of pain, while minimizing stiffness and maintaining motion. Surgical treatment of adult-acquired flatfoot may result in a variety of complications including recurrence of deformity as well as overcorrection of deformity with excessive stiffness and persistent pain.[9] Approaching the patient with recurrent deformity following a tendon transfer must be undertaken carefully as the tendency may be to introduce an element of overcorrection or resort to motion-sacrificing arthrodesis that may, in fact, be unnecessary. Either of these can result in significant stiffness of the foot and further dysfunction. In younger patients in particular, an effort to avoid motion-sacrificing arthrodesis due to its association with adjacent joint degeneration over time has a theoretical advantage. The focus of this article is to explore the approach to a recurrent flexible flatfoot deformity following failed primary tendon transfer, including the indications for arthrodesis.

EVALUATION OF RECURRENT DEFORMITY

Evaluation of the patient with recurrent deformity following tendon transfer for flexible deformity requires a detailed history and physical examination. In some cases, the evaluator may not have participated in the index surgical procedure. The authors recommend obtaining any previous operative reports if available as a clear understanding of the patient's complaints as well as the extent of the previous surgical procedure must be elucidated. The extent to which extra-articular corrections including either a medial displacement calcaneal osteotomy (MDCO), lateral column lengthening (LCL), or both were used to augment the medial soft tissue procedure and tendon transfer must be elucidated. The presence of a residual equinus deformity must also be recognized. Standing plain film radiographs including anteroposterior (AP) and lateral films of the foot with an AP film of the ankle are required to evaluate the radiographic alignment of the foot. Obtaining prior radiographs may be helpful to evaluate whether the index procedures failed due to undercorrection of the initial deformity. Magnetic resonance imaging may be helpful to more clearly evaluate the integrity of the medial soft tissues including the PTT and the tendon transfer. Particularly in patients with recurrence of deformity following limited arthrodesis or LCL, a computed tomography scan may be helpful to evaluate for nonunion resulting in collapse.

MEDIAL DISPLACEMENT CALCANEAL OSTEOTOMY IN THE TREATMENT OF RECURRENT DEFORMITY

A flexor digitorum longus (FDL) transfer with PTT debridement with or without advancement is occasionally utilized in the treatment of stage I and early stage II deformities. Although tendon transfer used in isolation to address flatfoot deformity may demonstrate satisfactory relief of pain at short-term follow-up, it does not address the biomechanical changes in flatfoot deformity. Eventually, it will fail leading to recurrence of pain and functional limitations.[6,7]

In patients developing progressive deformity following tendon transfer alone but without significant medial soft tissue attenuation and midfoot collapse resulting in forefoot abduction, an MDCO may be appropriate to augment the transfer. A gastrocnemius-soleus recession is also indicated if the patient has an equinus deformity. Den Hartog provided a nice explanation of the role for corrective osteotomy of the calcaneus in reinforcing a relatively weak FDL tendon transfer.[7] Medialization of the heel and pull of the Achilles complex facilitate hindfoot inversion following initiation of the PTT.[13,14] Additionally, improved gait parameters have been demonstrated following treatment of a flexible flatfoot deformity with MDCO and FDL transfer.[15] Primary restoration of an arch is not the goal of this procedure; improvement of hindfoot inversion through more favorable biomechanics of the Achilles and PTT results in improved gait mechanics, alleviation of pain, and preservation of hindfoot motion.

Hindfoot alignment may be addressed in part with an MDCO and FDL transfer; however, the procedure is not powerful enough to correct significant midfoot deformity. Patients do not typically report improvement in their arch height following MDCO coupled with FDL transfer. Despite pain relief in 97% of their patient population, Myerson and colleagues reported that only 87% of their study population thoughtt there was an improvement in their arch.[5] Guyton and colleagues similarly reported only 50% of their patient population reported an improvement in arch height.[8] Radiographic assessment and clinical improvement do not appear to correlate with patients' self-reported assessment of their arch height. Significant deformity including recurrence of forefoot abduction may necessitate additional procedures to adequately address the patient's symptoms.

LATERAL COLUMN LENGTHENING IN THE TREATMENT OF RECURRENT DEFORMITY

Particularly in younger patients failing primary MDCO with FDL transfer but with evidence of progressive flexible deformity and forefoot abduction, the surgeon should consider additional extra-articular correction in the form of an LCL and medial soft tissue reconstruction with spring ligament repair. Initially described by Evans, the LCL represents a powerful corrective extra-articular procedure for restoring the medial longitudinal arch, decreasing forefoot abduction, and hindfoot valgus associated with progressive flexible flatfoot deformity.[12,16,17] The technique is distinctly more powerful than an MDCO with FDL transfer in isolation with regard to deformity correction. The tendency, particularly in a revision situation, is to overcorrect the deformity leading to lateral column overload and persistent pain. Benthien and colleagues evaluated lateral column pressures in a cadaveric flatfoot model following LCL with a simulated FDL transfer.[18] Significant improvement compared to the severe flatfoot deformity was appreciated; however, lateral column pressures were also significantly increased. The addition of a medial cuneiform osteotomy restored lateral column pressures to values comparable to the intact foot model. Clinically, several authors have described increased lateral column pressures resulting in the development of calcaneocuboid arthrosis at mid- and long-term follow-up of unclear clinical significance.[6] Preexisting calcaneocuboid arthritis does not appear to be a contraindication to LCL. Persistent pain resulting from calcaneocuboid arthritis can be addressed with an isolated calcaneocuboid fusion, which does not appear to have a significant impact on subtalar motion.[6,9]

In an effort to avoid overcorrection, the senior author advocates meticulous evaluation of the correction, not only clinically but also under live fluoroscopic guidance intraoperatively. After creating an osteotomy in the calcaneus 10 to 12 mm proximal to the calcaneocuboid joint, a Hinterman retractor or lamina spreader can be used to serially distract the lateral column through the osteotomy while observing the degree of forefoot abduction (particularly talonavicular

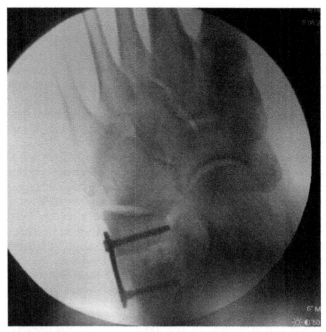

Fig. 1. Intraoperative fluoroscopic view following fixation of LCL is necessary to avoid overcorrection of forefoot abduction and increased lateral column overload.

coverage) under live fluoroscopy. Excessive forefoot adduction can be more readily avoided with this technique (**Fig. 1**). Both tricortical autograft and allograft have been effective in LCL[12,17]; the authors prefer a tricortical allograft that can be contoured to fit the osteotomy, which typically does not exceed 10 mm in width. Minimal fixation is needed; usually a low-profile 2-hole nonlocking plate is sufficient to stabilize the construct and minimize soft tissue irritation.[12,17]

When LCL is used as salvage for recurrent deformity in the flexible flatfoot, the authors recommend reevaluating the medial soft tissues including the PTT, the spring ligament, and the previous tendon transfer. A severely tendonotic PTT must be considered as a potential secondary pain generator if it was initially left intact at its insertion. Resection of the PTT may be indicated in this situation. The integrity of the tendon transfer should be evaluated. The authors prefer a short harvest technique with fixation in the navicular using a dorsal-to-plantar interference screw.[19] An attenuated FDL transfer is typically associated with insufficient correction of the deformity in the authors' experience. It is, therefore, particularly important to adequately address any residual deformity. The attenuated FDL tendon can be advanced; in rare cases when the previous FDL transfer was deemed ineffective and not amenable to advancement, the authors have transferred the FHL tendon to the navicular to augment the reconstruction. Following either debridement of the PTT or PTT resection, the presence or absence of a tear in the spring ligament can be directly visualized. In the event a tear is appreciated, the spring ligament is imbricated in a pants-over-vest fashion with suture. Despite literature suggesting double calcaneal osteotomy with medial soft tissue reconstruction may predispose to lateral column overload,[6,9,12,16,17] these techniques represent an effective motion-preserving approach for addressing recurrent deformity in the flexible flatfoot following tendon

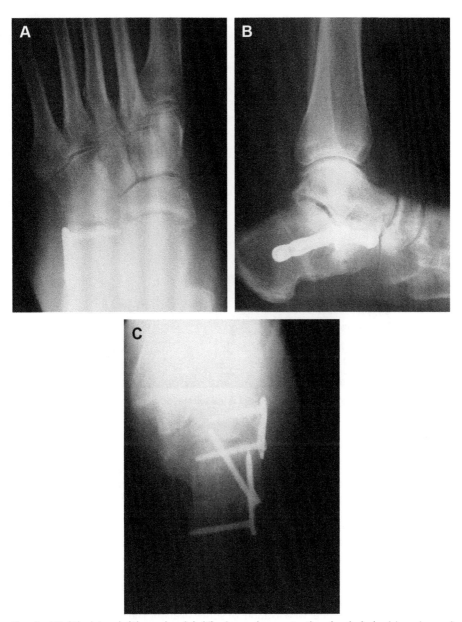

Fig. 2. AP (*A*), lateral (*B*), and axial (*C*) views demonstrating healed double calcaneal osteotomy with FDL transfer.

transfer (**Fig. 2**). Avoiding overcorrection, particularly with the LCL, is critical to ensure a successful outcome.

COTTON OSTEOTOMY FOR RESIDUAL FOREFOOT VARUS

A medial column procedure may be necessary to balance residual forefoot varus appreciated following joint-sparing procedures in the hindfoot. Unrecognized residual

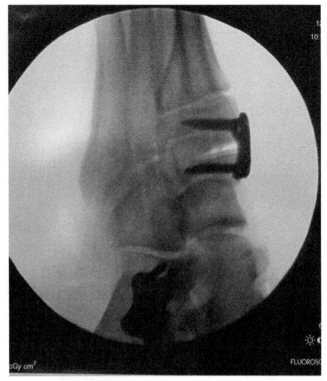

Fig. 3. Residual forefoot varus is readily addressed with a joint-sparing medial cuneiform or Cotton osteotomy.

fixed forefoot varus can contribute to failure of surgical intervention for a flexible flatfoot deformity. A medial cuneiform opening wedge osteotomy or Cotton osteotomy is an effective way to address residual forefoot varus deformity.[20] Although limited medial column fusions including a plantarflexion first tarsometatarsal joint fusion procedure have been described, in the absence of medial column arthritis, the authors prefer the Cotton osteotomy. The Cotton osteotomy provides a joint-sparing option for plantarflexion of the first ray. An assessment of the forefoot alignment including residual fixed forefoot varus should follow correction of the hindfoot; if necessary, the surgeon can readily perform the Cotton osteotomy. Fixation options are numerous and include obtaining an interference fit with an allograft of autograft without hardware, Kirschner wire fixation, or screw fixation. The authors prefer fixation with a dorsal plate (**Fig. 3**).

LIMITED HINDFOOT ARTHRODESIS IN THE TREATMENT OF RECURRENT DEFORMITY

The authors' preferred approach to recurrent stage II deformity has been clearly described here. A double calcaneal osteotomy with medial soft tissue reconstruction including PTT debridement or tenotomy, FDL transfer, and spring ligament repair if necessary is almost always preferable to hindfoot arthrodesis. However, some authors advocate a variety of limited hindfoot arthrodesis procedures in both the primary treatment of more severe flexible flatfoot deformities and the treatment of recurrent deformity.[4,6,9,10,21–23] Although there may be a theoretical advantage to motion-preserving options in an effort to preserve as much normal joint mechanics, occasionally, certain patient factors such as preexisting degenerative joint changes, morbid obesity, or severe medial soft tissue incompetence may make a limited hindfoot fusion a more predictable and technically easier procedure. Obesity is not a contraindication to joint-preserving procedures for flexible flatfoot deformity; however, limited hindfoot arthrodesis may be more appropriate in these patients as a primary procedure due to the higher risk of deformity recurrence following joint-preserving procedures. Certainly, failure of joint-preserving procedures in obese patients is a strong indication for limited hindfoot arthrodesis.

Realignment subtalar joint arthrodesis has been previously described as a primary treatment for stage II flatfoot deformity or as a salvage procedure for motion-preserving extra-articular procedures.[3,6] Realignment subtalar joint arthrodesis is a technically straightforward procedure with very predictable union rates, with some authors reporting rates approaching 100%.[3] The impact on hindfoot motion is marked but limited by preserved motion in the transverse tarsal joints. Following subtalar joint arthrodesis, talonavicular joint motion and calcaneocuboid motion are decreased 75% and 45%, respectively.[3,6,10] In the treatment of recurrent flatfoot deformity, a realignment subtalar joint arthrodesis provides a direct means of correcting hindfoot valgus and stabilizing the transverse tarsal joints while alleviating the pain associated with flexible flatfoot deformity, particularly subfibular impingement pain in the sinus tarsi. This is, of course, at the expense of hindfoot motion and with the relative risk of progressive adjacent joint degeneration at long-term follow-up.

Isolated talonavicular joint arthrodesis has been previously described for the treatment of a variety of hindfoot deformities including flexible flatfoot.[21,22] Its role in the correction of recurrent deformity has not been well elucidated. The literature suggests it is effective for decreasing pain and improving functional outcomes in adult flatfoot.[11,21] Harper reported 86% good or excellent results in 25 of 29 patients at an average follow-up of 26 months following isolated talonavicular arthrodesis.[22] In contrast to realignment subtalar joint arthrodesis, talonavicular arthrodesis sacrifices considerably more hindfoot motion resulting in an 80% decrease in hindfoot motion.[6] Therefore, with greater impairment of hindfoot motion, there is a more significant risk of progressive adjacent joint degeneration, which may have little impact in an elderly, low-demand patient, but discourages these authors from considering it among the primary revision procedures in the younger, more active individuals.

SUMMARY

Recurrent deformity in the adult flatfoot following previous tendon transfer represents a challenging treatment dilemma for even the most experienced foot and ankle surgeon. The evaluation must be comprehensive, resulting in a clear understanding of the extent to which previous surgical procedures either failed to address the deformity initially or led to progressive recurrence. Particularly in younger, more high-demand patients, every effort to preserve normal joint mechanics while alleviating pain and restoring functional alignment must be made. LCL coupled with MDCO and a comprehensive medial soft tissue reconstruction represents a joint-sparing modality for approaching even the most challenging flexible flatfoot deformities. Care to avoid overcorrection, particularly with a double calcaneal osteotomy, must be taken. In the presence of progressive degenerative changes or patient factors such as morbid obesity and advanced age, hindfoot arthrodesis, particularly realignment subtalar joint arthrodesis, provides a technically straightforward, predictable means of achieving a pain-free plantigrade foot. Talonavicular arthrodesis and double arthrodesis, although reliable means of achieving pain relief and functional alignment, do sacrifice considerably more hindfoot motion and are likely more appropriately reserved for elderly, low-demand patients or those with more severe fixed deformities.

REFERENCES

1. Johnson KA, Strom DE. Tibialis posterior tendon dysfunction. Clin Orthop 1989;239: 197–206.
2. Giza E, Cush G, Schon LC. The flexible flatfoot in the adult. Foot Ankle Clin 2007; 12(2):251–71.
3. Cohen BE, Johnson JE. Subtalar arthrodesis for treatment of posterior tibial tendon insufficiency. Foot Ankle Clin 2001;6(1):121–8.
4. Deland JT. Adult-acquired flatfoot deformity. J Am Acad Orthop Surg 2008;16(7): 399–406.
5. Myerson MS, Badekas A, Schon LC. Treatment of stage II posterior tibial tendon deficiency with flexor digitorum longus transfer and calcaneal osteotomy. Foot Ankle Int 2004;25(7):445–50.
6. Mosier-LaClair S, Pomeroy G, Manoli II A. Operative treatment of the difficult stage 2 adult acquired flatfoot deformity. Foot Ankle Clin 2001;6(1):95–119.
7. Den Hartog BD. Flexor digitorum longus transfer with medial displacement calcaneal osteotomy: biomechanical rationale. Foot Ankle Clin 2001;6(1):67–76.
8. Guyton GP, Jeng C, Krieger LE, et al. Flexor digitorum longus transfer and medial displacement calcaneal osteotomy for posterior tibial tendon dysfunction: a middle-term clinical follow-up. Foot Ankle Int 2001;22(8):627–32.
9. Neufeld SK, Myerson MS. Complications of surgical treatments for adult flatfoot deformities. Foot Ankle Clin 2001;6(1):179–91.
10. O'Malley MJ, Deland JT, Lee KT. Selective hindfoot arthrodesis for the treatment of adult acquired flatfoot deformity: an in vitro study. Foot Ankle Int 1995;16(7):411–7.
11. Fortin PT. Posterior tibial tendon insufficiency: isolated fusion of the talonavicular joint. Foot Ankle Clin 2001;6(1):137–51.
12. Philbin TM, Pokabla C, Berlet GC. Lateral column lengthening using allograft interposition and cervical plate fixation. Foot Ankle Spec 2008;1(5):288–96.
13. Nyska M, Parks BG, Chu IT, et al. The contribution of the medial calcaneal osteotomy to the correction of flatfoot deformities. Foot Ankle Int 2001;22(4):278–82.
14. Hadfield MH, Snyder JW, Liacouras PC, et al. Effects of medializing calcaneal osteotomy on Achilles tendon lengthening and plantar foot pressures. Foot Ankle Int 2003;24(7):523–9.
15. Brodsky JW, Charlick DA, Coleman SC, et al. Hindfoot motion following reconstruction for posterior tibial tendon dysfunction. Foot Ank Int 2009;30(7):613–8.
16. Sangeorzan BJ, Mosca V, Hansen Jr ST. Effect of calcaneal lengthening on relationships among hindfoot, midfoot, and forefoot. Foot Ankle 1993;14(3):136–41.
17. Dolan CM, Henning JA, Anderson JG, et al. randomized prospective study comparing tri-cortical iliac crest autograft to allograft in the lateral column lengthening component for operative correction of adult acquired flatfoot deformity. Foot Ankle Int 2007;28(1): 8–12.
18. Benthien RA, Parks BG, Guyton GP, et al. Lateral column calcaneal lengthening, flexor digitorum longus transfer, and opening wedge medial calcaneal osteotomy for flexible flatfoot: a biomechanical study. Foot Ankle Int 2007;28(1):70–7.
19. Bussewitz BW, Hyer CF. Interference screw fixation and short harvest using flexor digitorum longus (FDL) transfer for posterior tibial tendon dysfunction: a technique. J Foot Ankle Surg 2010;49:501–3.

20. Tankson CJ. The Cotton osteotomy: indications and techniques. Foot Ankle Clin 2007;12:309–15.
21. Crevoisier X. The isolated talonavicular arthrodesis. Foot Ankle Clin 2011;16(1): 49–59.
22. Harper MC. Talonavicular arthrodesis for the acquired flatfoot in the adult. Clin Orthop Relat Res 1999;365:65–8.
23. Thelen S, Rutt J, Wild M, et al. The influence of talonavicular versus double arthrodesis on load dependent motion of the midtarsal joint. Arch Orthop Trauma Surg 2010; 130(1):47–53.

Management of the Rigid Arthritic Flatfoot in Adults: Triple Arthrodesis

Jamal Ahmad, MD*, David Pedowitz, MS, MD

KEYWORDS

- Arthritis • Calcaneocuboid • Double • Rigid flatfoot • Subtalar • Talonavicular
- Triple arthrodesis

KEY POINTS

- The traditional surgical treatment for the rigid arthritic flatfoot (AAFD) is a triple arthrodesis of the subtalar (ST), talonavicular (TN), and calcaneocuboid (CC) joints through a combined lateral and medial approach.
- The triple arthrodesis is highly successful in correcting deformity, alleviating pain, and improving function.
- After triple arthrodesis, patients can develop either early or late postoperative difficulties.
- Alternatives to the dual-incision triple arthrodesis include a single medial approach to the triple arthrodesis, a double arthrodesis of the TN and CC joints, and a modified double arthrodesis of the ST and TN joints.
- Further study is needed to define the role of alternate approaches and arthrodeses in managing the rigid, AAFD.

Appropriate management of the adult flatfoot deformity (AAFD) is highly dependent upon its severity. Upon failure of nonsurgical treatment, patients with a flexible flatfoot and no arthritic changes are amenable to soft-tissue reconstruction and bony osteotomies that correct deformity and preserve joints. Once adults develop a rigid, arthritic flatfoot, however, such joint-sparing procedures are neither appropriate nor sufficient. The traditional surgical treatment for the rigid arthritic flatfoot that has failed nonoperative management is a triple arthrodesis of the subtalar (ST), talonavicular (TN), and calcaneocuboid (CC) joints through a combined lateral and medial approach.

Ryerson[1] first described this dual-incision triple arthrodesis in 1923 as treatment of a rigid deformity secondary to paralytic conditions. As these types of diseases

Rothman Institute Orthopaedics, Thomas Jefferson University Hospital, 925 Chestnut Street, Philadelphia, PA 19107, USA
* Corresponding author.
E-mail address: jamal.ahmad@rothmaninstitute.com

Foot Ankle Clin N Am 17 (2012) 309–322
http://dx.doi.org/10.1016/j.fcl.2012.03.008
1083-7515/12/$ – see front matter © 2012 Elsevier Inc. All rights reserved.

foot.theclinics.com

became less common and more of a historical significance, the triple arthrodesis was adapted to address the rigid arthritic adult flatfoot.[2,3] To date, this procedure is highly successful in correcting deformity and relieving both mechanical and arthritic pain.[4,5] However, the triple arthrodesis is not without shortcomings. Early and late postoperative problems include lateral wound complications, malunion, nonunion, and adjacent joint arthritis.[6-9] Several modifications in the traditional technique of triple arthrodesis have recently been proposed to overcome these difficulties. Such alterations include the use of a single medial incision, exclusion of the ST or CC joint, and greater inclusion of the medial column of the midfoot.[10-12]

TRIPLE ARTHRODESIS
Surgical Indications

The triple arthrodesis is indicated as the traditional surgical treatment for the rigid, arthritic AAFD.[13] Whether owing to posttraumatic arthritis or advanced posterior tibial tendon dysfunction, it is ideally suited for addressing both deformity and arthritis of the ST, TN, and CC joints. This procedure is contraindicated in patients with a poor soft-tissue envelope or vascular status of the hindfoot that would endanger wound healing.

Preoperative Planning

Preoperative planning for the triple arthrodesis begins with a thorough history taking and physical examination of the patient. Special attention should be paid to patient factors that can affect bone and wound healing. These include medical conditions such as diabetes and inflammatory arthropathy, medications such as steroids and non-steroidal anti-inflammatory drugs, and social factors like tobacco usage. Upon patient examination, the rigidity of the flatfoot must be confirmed. Particular attention should be paid to the alignment of the hindfoot, whether there is an equinus contracture of the ankle, and if rigid forefoot varus is a contributing factor in the deformity. In addition, the patient's soft-tissue and vascular condition should be assessed and deemed appropriate for surgical treatment.

Weight-bearing radiographs of the foot in the anteroposterior, lateral, and oblique planes are most important in planning a triple arthrodesis. Weight-bearing films allow for more accurate evaluation of malalignment and loss of joint space.[14] Close attention should be paid to the apex of the flatfoot deformity on the lateral radiograph. Arch collapse can develop at the TN, naviculocuneiform (NC), tarsometatarsal joints, or any combination thereof. To provide the most appropriate surgical treatment, the surgeon should be aware of the precise location of the patient's deformity. It is also important to assess the ankle for its possible involvement in the rigid flatfoot with weight-bearing radiographs in the anteroposterior, lateral, and mortise planes. If the ankle also displays rigid deformity and/or arthritis, then a triple arthrodesis is insufficient for complete treatment.[15] Rather, the patient may require an arthrodesis that includes the ankle joint, which is outside the scope of this chapter (**Fig. 1**).[16,17]

The alignment of the whole leg needs to be assessed because this may affect the final positioning of the proposed triple arthrodesis. If there is a history of prior limb trauma, full-length limb radiographs may be required. At the very least, the tibial alignment should be ascertained in all cases.

Traditional Operative Technique

Currently, the traditional surgical exposure for a triple arthrodesis is a combined lateral and medial approach.[18] The lateral incision begins at the distal end of the

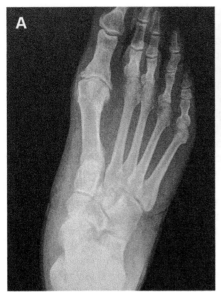
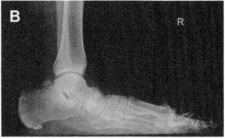

Fig. 1. (*A, B*) Preoperative radiographs of an adult patient with a rigid flatfoot deformity. Note the degenerative changes at the ST, TN, and CC joints that accompany the planovalgus deformity.

lateral malleolus and extends to the base of the fourth metatarsal. The muscle belly of the extensor digitorum brevis is isolated superior to the peroneal tendons and elevated to visualize the CC joint. The sinus tarsi is thoroughly debrided at the proximal end of this incision to expose the ST joint. The medial incision begins at the medial malleolus and extends to the NC joint. A plane is created between the distal PTT and anterior tibial tendons to visualize the TN joint. There are no major vulnerable neurovascular structures that cross this plane and it is a relatively safe exposure.

Once all 3 joints have been exposed, their osteophytes and diseased articular cartilage are removed to expose subchondral bone. Various instruments that can be used for this purpose include a micro-oscillating sagittal saw, chisels, and/or curettes. If curettes are to be used, drilling of the cartilage with a guide pin may be necessary to fenestrate and debride particularly sclerotic areas. Care should be taken to avoid excess bony resection and shortening of the foot.

Once the joints are properly prepared, they can be mobilized sequentially to correct the patient's rigid flatfoot deformity. This begins with the ST joint as it is reduced and fixed in 0° to 5° of valgus. ST fixation is achieved with 1 or 2 partially threaded, cannulated cancellous screws of at least 6.5 mm in diameter.[19] These can be placed either starting from plantar calcaneus through the talar body or vice versa.[20] It is important to note that there is no current consensus among surgeons with regard to the specific number, size, and direction of screws to use.[21,22] The first and second authors' preferences are to respectively use a single 6.5- or 7.0-mm partially threaded cannulated screw from the posterior, inferior calcaneus toward the central talar body.

The TN joint is reduced next with combined inversion of the transverse tarsal joints and plantarflexion of the first ray. This specific realignment maneuver restores the windlass mechanism and arch shape of the foot.[23,24] A wide variety of materials have been utilized to achieve TN arthrodesis. Such devices include cannulated compression screws, staples, plate and screw constructs, and a combination thereof.[25-27] The difficulty with TN arthrodesis fixation in particular is 2-fold. The apposing surfaces are curved in both the coronal and sagittal plane, making preparation arduous. In addition, the starting point for most screws is the tuberosity, which is far medial from the central axis of the joint and makes compression of the more central and lateral joint surfaces difficult to achieve. There are a few biomechanical studies that compare different types of TN implants, but no single device has a proven advantage over another.[28] The first author's preference is to use two, 4.5-mm, partially threaded, cannulated cancellous screws in a distal-to-proximal direction. The second author routinely uses a compression staple plate across the TN joint dorsally and additional fixation with a single cannulated screw starting in the tuberosity passed into the talar body.

Finally, any flatfoot deformity that remains is corrected through arthrodesis of the CC joint. Upon ST and TN realignment and fusion, the space at the CC joint is carefully assessed. If there is minimal persistent flatfoot deformity and/or gapping at the CC joint, it can be fused in situ. However, this cannot be done if there is significant residual deformity and/or space at the joint. Rather, the CC joint must be addressed through an arthrodesis with interpositional bone graft to provide simultaneous bony apposition, lateral column lengthening, and complete deformity correction.[29] In situations where the CC joint requires this type of distraction arthrodesis, consideration should be given to performing this before addressing the TN joint. Akin to the TN joint, CC arthrodesis can be achieved with a wide variety of devices. Such implants include screws, staples, or a plate and screw construct.[30,31] To date, different implants have only been compared with regard to providing a distraction CC arthrodesis. Kimball and associates[32] found a plate and screw construct to have a significantly higher stiffness and load to failure than cortical screws in a biomechanical study. The first author's preference is to use compression staples or a 4-hole lateral column lengthening plate to perform an in situ or distraction CC arthrodesis respectively. The second author routinely uses a compression staple plate for the CC joint (**Fig. 2**).

After the triple arthrodesis is complete, the foot should be assessed for any persistent deformity. If patients have contracture of the gastrocnemius muscle or Achilles tendon, an additional Strayer recession or Achilles lengthening is performed, respectively.[33] Residual forefoot varus can be managed either with an opening-wedge Cotton osteotomy of the medial cuneiform or a tarsometatarsal arthrodesis.[34,35] The choice of midfoot procedures is dependent upon midfoot rigidity and/or arthritis and is outside the scope of this article.

The use of adjuvant bone graft during a triple arthrodesis remains controversial. For patients with minimal deformity, the subchondral bone requires minimal resection and graft may not be necessary to achieve bony apposition at any of the 3 joints. Rosenfeld and co-workers[36] performed 100 triple arthrodeses with local bone graft from resected subchondral bone. With a reported nonunion rate as low as 4%, they conclude that bone grafting is not needed in most situations. However, it is important to recognize that the lateral column of the foot can shorten with a severe enough deformity.[37] Treating this situation requires bone grafting to lengthen the lateral column, completely correct the deformity, and achieve a plantigrade foot. Graft options vary between morcellized and structural wedge allografts and autografts.[38] The most commonly used sources of autograft are the iliac crest, proximal tibia, and distal tibia.[39-41] To date, there are limited studies that compare the use of allograft, autograft, and no bone graft when a triple arthrodesis is performed. McGarvey and

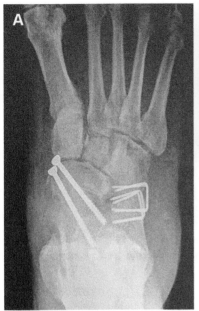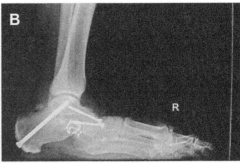

Fig. 2. (*A, B*) Postoperative radiographs of a patient who underwent a triple arthrodesis. Prior deformity has been corrected through careful joint preparation and rigid internal fixation.

Braly[42] performed a nonrandomized, retrospective study on 24 and 17 patients who received iliac crest autografts and allografts with their triple arthrodesis, respectively.[42] More nonunions were seen in the allograft (3 of 24 [12.5%]) than the autograft (1 of 17 [5.9%]) population. However, this difference was not found to be significant. For primary arthrodesis, the first and second authors use morcellized and structural allograft for minimal and severe deformities, respectively. Both authors reserve iliac crest autograft for revision arthrodesis. In the event that a patient may require treatment of a future ankle condition, some consideration should be given to avoiding harvesting bone graft from the distal tibia.

Postoperatively, patients are immobilized and rendered non–weight-bearing until bony healing becomes evident on radiographs. This typically occurs at 6 to 8 weeks from surgery.[43] At this point, patients are allowed progressive weight-bearing in a fracture boot or walking cast until bony fusion is complete. The time to achieve full healing is typically between 3 and 6 months.[44]

Although there is much literature with long-term follow-up regarding the traditional 2-incision triple arthrodesis, it is important to distinguish early from recent studies. Early research described outcomes in which the procedure was performed with absent or minimal internal fixation. Saltzman and associates[45] examined long-term outcomes in 57 patients with 67 triple arthrodeses. Whereas most patients had significant pain improvement, 78% had some recurrence of deformity and 19% developed a nonunion of the fusion, with the TN joint affected the most.

Over the past decade, more literature has been published that examines operative outcomes with the use of modern, rigid internal fixation. These more recent studies predictably describe better results. In one of the larger and more current studies, Pell

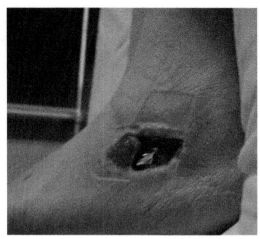

Fig. 3. Patient who developed a deep lateral wound dehiscence after a triple arthrodesis with a distraction CC fusion. The wound healed with surgical debridement and vacuum-assisted closure.

and colleagues[4] conducted medium and long-term follow-up on 111 patients with a rigid, arthritic flatfoot. They reported rates of maintaining deformity correction, patient satisfaction, and bony union to be higher than 90%. More recently, Czurda and associates[46] performed medium-term follow-up on a smaller population of 20 patients. Although 25% of their patients reported some residual pain, the authors observed that all patients had improvement in pain, function, and deformity with no occurrence of nonunion. Child and colleagues[47] also performed a medium-term study in 24 patients, but focused on correlations between correction of radiographic deformity and change in symptoms. They found the triple arthrodesis to be highly reliable and reproducible in correcting a rigid flatfoot deformity. They also found improvement in symptoms to be greatest when the flatfoot was realigned closest to a normal shape.

With regard to adverse events after a triple arthrodesis, it is important to distinguish between those that occur in the short term versus the long term. The most common acute or subacute problems that have been reported are wound complications, malunion, and nonunion. Wound healing problems have been noted in 2% to 25% of patients, with the higher range of this incidence occurring in patients with rheumatoid arthritis. The majority of reported wound complications is superficial and affects the lateral incision. The lateral wound is at greater risk for problems, because its skin and soft tissue may be placed under tension with flatfoot deformity correction as the midfoot is adducted to correct the common midfoot abduction deformity. Malunion has been reported to occur in as many as 4% of patients. Maenpaa and associates[6] found that half of malunited patients had undercorrection, whereas the other half displayed overcorrection of deformity. Although all of these patients had rheumatoid arthritis, the authors attributed most of these malunions to be owing to surgeon errors and the inherent complexity of the procedure. Among all short-term complications, nonunion after arthrodesis is the most reported. Observed rates of nonunion range between 2 and 13%, with the TN joint being affected the most **(Fig. 3)**.[48]

Even after the triple arthrodesis is fully healed, patients may develop dysfunction in the long term. Several authors make note of significant limitations with walking inclines, accommodating uneven ground, and stair climbing.[49] Formal gait studies after triple arthrodesis show decreased ankle dorsiflexion, cadence, and stride with decreased midfoot motion. Gait and function are further affected if patients develop adjacent joint arthritis. Smith and co-workers[5] followed patients for 15 years after surgery and found that 27% of patients with a triple arthrodesis had developed symptomatic adjacent joint arthritis in the ankle, NC, and/or tarsometatarsal joints. De Groot and associates[50] examined only radiographs after triple arthrodesis and found adjacent joint arthritis in 47% of patients at 10-year follow-up. This occurs likely because of the increased demands on the foot and ankle with the ST, TN, and CC joints fused. All these problems can worsen if a triple arthrodesis is performed on patients with bilateral rigid flatfeet. To date, there is scant literature regarding how patients function with a bilateral triple arthrodesis. However, it is logical to reason that a bilateral triple arthrodesis can be as limiting to a patient, if not more so, than a unilateral fusion. To date, many authors have acknowledged surgical outcomes that improve within the intermediate term and then deteriorate by long-term follow-up.[51] Raikin[52] described the triple arthrodesis as a "salvage procedure" in which gait dysfunction and adjacent joint arthritis should be considered an expected sequelae rather than a failure of the procedure. Although the triple arthrodesis is a valid treatment option for the rigid and/or arthritic flatfoot, its risks and consequences cannot be ignored.

Single Incision Triple Arthrodesis

In an effort to minimize wound complications from the traditional dual-incision surgical approach, some surgeons have attempted the triple arthrodesis through a single incision. Bono and co-workers[53] utilized a single lateral incision in a cadaver model to determine the amount of cartilage that could be removed from the ST, TN, and CC joints. They report that, although they were able to debride cartilage and subchondral bone from 80% of the ST and 90% of the CC joint, only 38% of cartilage could be removed from the TN joint. The authors attributed the difficulty with preparing the TN joint to inadequate visualization of the talar head. They recommended performing the TN arthrodesis through a medial incision and concluded that an appropriate triple arthrodesis could not be conducted through a single lateral approach.

After such cadaveric studies, the single incision approach to the triple arthrodesis has since been attempted only from the medial side. Akin to Bono and associates,[53] Jeng and colleagues[54] evaluated the quantity of articular cartilage that could be debrided from the ST, TN, and CC joints through a single medial incision in cadavers. To obtain both medial and lateral joint exposure from a single medial incision, the authors admit to making some modifications in technique from the medial approach of a traditional triple arthrodesis. Before starting the medial incision, they percutaneously released the peroneal tendons to relieve longstanding contracture from the hindfoot valgus component of deformity. Akin to the traditional triple arthrodesis, the medial incision that Jeng and co-workers make is still from the medial malleolus to the NC joint to expose the TN joint. However, the authors perform increased soft-tissue dissection to visualize the ST joint. Then, they increasingly distracted the TN joint to expose the CC joint. With this technique, they report that they were able to expose and remove greater than or equal to 90% of articular cartilage from all 3 joints. Unlike a single lateral surgical exposure, they conclude that the medial approach allows adequate and comparable access to all 3 joints for a triple arthrodesis.

Although these results are promising, there are limited clinical studies regarding a single medial incision to perform a triple arthrodesis. After their cadaveric work, Jeng and co-workers[55] performed 17 triple arthrodeses through a single medial incision with final follow-up at an average of 3.5 years postoperatively. No patients developed wound healing problems. Although all patients achieved ST and TN arthrodesis, CC fusion was incomplete in 2 of the 17 patients (both with an asymptomatic pseudo-arthrosis). It is important to recognize that using only a medial incision may have limited the authors' ability to fuse the CC joint. Although they were able to place ST and TN implants through the medial incision directly, CC implants had to be limited to screws that were placed percutaneously. Despite this shortcoming, Jeng and associates concluded that the medial approach to triple arthrodesis was a reliable technique with outcomes comparable to the standard dual-incision triple arthrodesis. Although this single incision for a triple arthrodesis does avoid lateral wound complications and may hold promise as an alternative technique, additional data are required to determine its future role in treatment.

DOUBLE ARTHRODESIS (TN AND CC)

As stated, the triple arthrodesis has been the traditional surgical treatment for the rigid, arthritic AAFD despite observed long-term complications. Certainly, if the ST, TN, and CC joints are all arthritic, a triple arthrodesis cannot be avoided. Over the past decade, there has been interest in fusing fewer joints to attain the same deformity correction while avoiding problems like adjacent joint arthritis. If the AAFD is rigid but 1 joint can be spared owing to minimal arthritic changes, a double arthrodesis may be a viable treatment option. To date, there has been less certainty in the historical literature and common jargon as to which joints are involved when referring to a double arthrodesis, or "double" as it is often shortened. In 1959, DuVries defined a "double" arthrodesis as a fusion of the TN and CC joints.[56] In more recent situations, a "double" has been used to describe a ST and TN arthrodesis.[57] With these circumstances in mind, the term "modified double" is used in this chapter for clarification of an ST and TN arthrodesis.

Compelling biomechanical data suggest that a double arthrodesis can effectively treat the rigid, arthritic AAFD when there is minimal ST arthritis. In a cadaver model, O'Malley and co-workers[58] assessed the ability to correct deformity with selective hindfoot arthrodeses. They found that although the ST, TN, and CC joints are interconnected, they differ in their contribution to deformity. In their study, an ST fusion did not achieve consistent deformity correction. However, they found that either a TN or double arthrodesis restored alignment in a flatfoot with considerable laxity through the transverse tarsal joints. Astion and colleagues[59] also examined the ST, TN, and CC joints in cadaveric specimens, but used a 3-dimensional magnetic space tracking system. They found that any combination of arthrodeses that included the TN joint limited motion at the remaining joint or joints to approximately 2° of motion.[59] In contrast, they found that exclusion of the TN joint from the arthrodesis resulted in considerable motion through the hindfoot. They concluded that the TN joint was the "key" to the triple joint complex and its fusion essentially eliminated motion at the other 2 joints. Using an ultrasonic motion system, similar results were obtained by Wülker and associates,[60] who found that ST motion was decreased by approximately 75% with TN fusion.

Clinical studies further support the role of a double arthrodesis in certain patients with rigid AAFD. Mann and Beaman[61] performed a 4-year follow-up on patients with double arthrodeses and found high rates of satisfaction (83%) and symptom relief (76%). The most common complication seen in this study was nonunion of the TN joint. Beischer and colleagues[62] performed a comparative study on patients who underwent either a triple or double at longer than 5 years postoperatively. They found

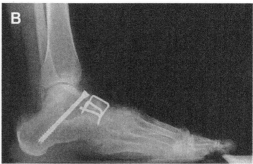

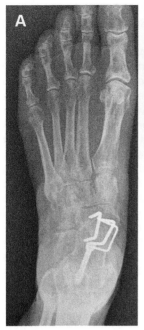

Fig. 4. (*A, B*) Patient with a double TN and CC arthrodesis. Note that there are no degenerative changes at the ST joint.

that both the triple or double arthrodesis were similar in providing decreased pain and increased function. Although this literature holds promise, it is important to realize that there are currently no studies with long-term follow-up of the double arthrodesis. It remains to be seen if this procedure can avoid some of the long-term dysfunction seen after a triple arthrodesis.

Both authors' experience with the double arthrodesis is similar to that of Mann and Beischer. Surgical indications are for patients with advanced flatfoot deformity without arthritic change at the ST joint. Both authors perform this through a dual-incision technique similar to the traditional triple arthrodesis. The fusion itself is achieved using compression "staple" type plates and additional interfragmentary compression screws across the arthrodesis site. If needed, this is combined with an Achilles lengthening or Strayer recession. Neither author routinely performs isolated TN arthrodeses because of the high biomechanical demands placed on that joint when correcting deformity.[63] Instead, the CC joint is added to the arthrodesis for further stability (**Fig. 4**).

MODIFIED DOUBLE ARTHRODESIS (ST AND TN)

When the rigid, arthritic AAFD includes ST arthritis, there is no debate that the ST joint should be included in the arthrodesis. However, if the CC joint has minimal degenerative changes, a modified double arthrodesis may offer a viable treatment option. The modified double can be performed either through combined medial and lateral incisions or a single medial approach. The dual-incision technique is the same as that used in a standard triple arthrodesis, with the exception that the lateral incision does not need to be extended distally to expose the CC joint. When performed through a single medial incision, the technique is similar to that described above for the single medial incision triple arthrodesis, with the exception that the CC joint need not be exposed.

Although literature is limited, the modified double arthrodesis has found success with both pain relief and deformity correction for certain patients with rigid AAFD. Knupp and associates[64] evaluated 32 modified double arthrodeses through a single medial approach at an average of 21 months and found a complete fusion in all patients at 13 weeks. Brilhault[65] reviewed 11 patients who underwent this procedure, performed primarily because they had a deficient or concerning lateral skin flap. At an average of 21.5 months postoperatively, he found that all patients had improvement in hindfoot alignment, pain, ambulation, and footwear requirements.[65] Sammarco and associates[66] achieved similar results in 16 patients at 18 months after a modified double arthrodesis. All patients were highly satisfied with improvements in pain, function, deformity, and return to desired shoe wear. All of these authors concluded that the modified double arthrodesis is a reasonable option for treating the rigid, arthritic AAFD in which the CC joint is relatively spared.

Although recent studies offer promise, it is important to realize that there are currently no studies with long-term follow-up of the modified double arthrodesis. Many surgeons who perform this procedure claim that it has several advantages over a triple arthrodesis. Because the CC joint is excluded from the fusion, the modified double arthrodesis has shorter operative times and eliminates any complications that could be attributed to a CC fusion such as nonunion. In preserving CC joint motion at the lateral column, it has been argued that patients should develop less long-term adjacent joint disease with a modified double than a triple arthrodesis. However, this particular advantage remains theoretical, because its supporting evidence is currently anecdotal. To date, there are no

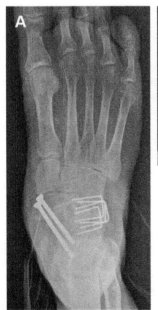
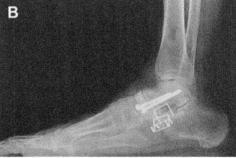

Fig. 5. (A, B) Patient with a double ST and TN arthrodesis. Note that there are no degenerative changes at the CC joint.

studies that compare outcomes of the modified double and triple arthrodesis. It remains to be seen if the modified double arthrodesis can avoid some of the long-term dysfunction seen after a triple arthrodesis (**Fig. 5**).

SUMMARY

The traditional surgical treatment for adults with a rigid, arthritic flatfoot is a dual-incision triple arthrodesis. Over time, this procedure has proved to be reliable and reproducible in obtaining successful deformity correction through fusion and good clinical results. However, the traditional dual-incision triple arthrodesis is not without shortcomings. Early complications include lateral wound problems, malunion, and nonunion. Long-term follow-up of patients after a triple arthrodesis has shown that many develop adjacent joint arthritis at the ankle or midfoot. This particular problem should be considered an expected consequence, rather than a failure of the procedure. Although the indications for and surgical techniques used in triple arthrodesis have evolved and improved with time (predictably improving results in the intermediate term), the triple arthrodesis should be regarded as a salvage procedure.

Certain measures can be taken by the surgeon to avoid some problems. If patients are at risk for lateral wound complications, the arthrodesis could be performed through a single medial incision. However, this can make some aspects of the CC fusion more difficult. Implants would have to be inserted percutaneously, which prevents the surgeon from using either staples or plates. If a patient were to need a lateral column lengthening through a CC distraction fusion, this would not be possible medially. If either the ST or CC joints have minimal degenerative changes, they could be spared through a double or modified double arthrodesis, respectively. Although these procedures that deviate from the traditional triple arthrodesis offer promise, further study is required to better define their role in treatment of the rigid, arthritic AAFD.

Triple arthrodesis is, by no means, a simple surgery. It requires preoperative planning, meticulous preparation of bony surfaces, cognizance of hindfoot position-ing, and rigidity of fixation. The procedure also requires enough experience on the part of the operating surgeon to anticipate postoperative problems and provide modifications in traditional technique for certain patients.

REFERENCES

1. Ryerson E. Arthrodesing operations on the feet. J Bone Joint Surg Am 1923;5: 453–71.
2. Wilson FC Jr, Fay GF, Lamotte P, et al. Triple arthrodesis: a study of the factors affecting fusion after three hundred and one procedures. J Bone Joint Surg Am 1965;47:340–8.
3. Duncan JW, Lovell WW. Hoke triple arthrodesis. J Bone Joint Surg Am 1978;60: 795–8.
4. Pell RF, Myerson MS, Schon LC. Clinical outcome after primary triple arthrodesis. J Bone Joint Surg Am 2000;82:47–57.
5. Smith RW, Shen W, DeWitt S, et al. Triple arthrodesis in adults with non-paralytic disease. J Bone Joint Surg Am 2004;86:2707–13.
6. Maenpaa H, Lehto MU, Belt EA. What went wrong in triple arthrodesis? An analysis of failures in 21 patients. Clin Orthop Relat Res 2001;391:218–23.
7. Figgie MP, O'Malley MJ, Ranawat C, et al. Triple arthrodesis in rheumatoid arthritis. Clin Orthop Relat Res 1993;292:250–4.
8. Knupp M, Skoog A, Tornkvist H, et al. Triple arthrodesis in rheumatoid arthritis. Foot Ankle Int 2008;29:293–7.

9. Doayan A, Albayrak M, Uayur F, et al. Triple arthrodesis in rigid foot deformities and the effect of internal fixation on clinical and radiographic results. Acta Orthop Traumatol Turc 2006;40:200–27.

10. Jeng CL, Vora AM, Myerson MS. The medial approach to triple arthrodesis. Indications and Technique for management of rigid valgus deformities in high-risk patients. Foot Ankle Clin North Am 2005;10:515–21.

11. Weinraub GM, Schuberth JM, Lee M, et al. Isolated medial incisional approach to subtalar and talonavicular arthrodesis. J Foot Ankle Surg 2010;49:326–30.

12. Barg A, Brunner S, Zwicky L, et al. Subtalar and naviculocuneiform fusion for extended breakdown of the medial arch. Foot Ankle Clin North Am 2011;16:69–81.

13. Bennett GL, Graham CE, Mauldin DM. Triple arthrodesis in adults. Foot Ankle Int 1991;12:138–43.

14. Wapner KL. Triple arthrodesis in adults. J Am Acad Orthop Surg 1998;6:188–96.

15. Bohay DR, Anderson JG. Stage IV posterior tibial tendon insufficiency: the tilted ankle. Foot Ankle Clin North Am 2006;12:619–36.

16. Acosta R, Ushiba J, Cracchiolo A. The results of a primary and staged pantalar arthrodesis and tibiotalocalcaneal arthrodesis in adult patients. Foot Ankle Int 2000; 21:182–94.

17. Kelly I, Nunley J. Treatment of stage 4 adult acquired flatfoot. Foot Ankle Clin North Am 2001;6:167–78.

18. Johnson JE, Yu JR. Arthrodesis techniques in the management of stage II and III acquired adult flatfoot deformity. J Bone Joint Surg Am 2005;87:1866–76.

19. Easley ME, Trnka HJ, Schon LC, et al. Isolated subtalar arthrodesis. J Bone Joint Surg Am 2000;82:613–24.

20. McGlamry MC, Robitaille MF. Analysis of screw pullout strength: a function of screw orientation in subtalar joint arthrodesis. J Foot Ankle Surg 2004;43:277–84.

21. Gosch C, Verrette R, Lindsey DP, et al. Comparison of initial compression force across the subtalar joint by two different screw fixation techniques. J Foot Ankle Surg 2006;45:168–73.

22. Lee JY, Lee JS. Optimal double screw configuration for subtalar arthrodesis: a finite element analysis. Knee Surg Sports Traumatol Arthrosc 2011;19:842–9.

23. Richie Jr DH. Biomechanics and clinical analysis of the adult acquired flatfoot. Clin Podiatr Med Surg 2007;24:617–44.

24. Giza E, Cush G, Schon LC. The flexible flatfoot in the adult. Foot Ankle Clin North Am 2007;12:251–71.

25. Harper MC. Talonavicular arthrodesis for the acquired flatfoot in the adult. Clin Orthop Relat Res 1999;365:65–8.

26. Chen CH, Huang PJ, Chen TB, et al. Isolated talonavicular arthrodesis for talonavicular arthrodesis. Foot Ankle Int 2001;22:633–8.

27. Weinraub GM, Heilala MA. Isolated talonavicular arthrodesis for adult onset flatfoot deformity/posterior tibial tendon dysfunction. Clin Podiatr Med Surg 2007;24:745–52.

28. Jarrell III SE, Owen JR, Wayne JS, et al. Biomechanical comparison of screw versus plate/screw construct for talonavicular fusion. Foot Ankle Int 2009;30:150–6.

29. Horton GA, Olney BW. Triple arthrodesis with lateral column lengthening for treatment of severe planovalgus deformity. Foot Ankle Int 1995;16:395–400.

30. Kann JN, Parks BG, Schon LC. Biomechanical evaluation of two different screw positions for fusion of the calcaneocuboid joint. Foot Ankle Int 1999;20:33–6.

31. Mereau TM, Ford TC. Nitinol compression staples for bone fixation in foot surgery. J Am Podiatr Med Assoc 2006;96:102–6.

32. Kimball HL, Aronow MS, Sullivan RJ, et al. Biomechanical evaluation of calcaneo-cuboid distraction arthrodesis: a cadaver study of two different fixation methods. Foot Ankle Int 2000;21:845–8.
33. DiGiovanni CW, Langer P. The role of isolated gastrocnemius and combined Achilles contractures in the flatfoot. Foot Ankle Clin North Am 2007;12:363–79.
34. Hirose CB, Johnson JE. Plantarflexion opening wedge medial cuneiform osteotomy for correction of fixed forefoot varus associated with flatfoot deformity. Foot Ankle Int 2004;28:568–74.
35. Thompson IM, Bohay DR, Anderson JG. Fusion rate of first tarsometatarsal arthrodesis in the modified Lapidus procedure and flatfoot reconstruction. Foot Ankle Int 2005;26:698–703.
36. Rosenfeld PF, Budgen SA, Saxby TS. Triple arthrodesis: is bone grafting necessary? The results in 100 consecutive cases. J Bone Joint Surg Br 2005;87:175–8.
37. Sands AK, Tansey JP. Lateral column lengthening. Foot Ankle Clin North Am 2007;12:301–8.
38. Neufeld SK, Uribe J, Myerson MS. Use of structural allograft to compensate for bone loss in arthrodesis of the foot and ankle. Foot Ankle Clin North Am 2002;7:1–17.
39. Fitzgibbons TC, Hawks MA, McMullen ST, et al. Bone grafting in surgery about the foot and ankle: indications and techniques. J Am Acad Orthop Surg 2011;19:112–20.
40. Whitehouse MR, Lankester BJ, Winson IG, et al. Bone graft harvest from the proximal tibia in foot and ankle arthrodesis surgery. Foot Ankle Int 2006;27:913–6.
41. Danzinger MB, Abdo RV, Decker JE. Distal tibia bone graft for arthrodesis of the foot and ankle. Foot Ankle Int 1995;16:187–90.
42. McGarvey WC, Braly WG. Bone graft in hindfoot arthrodesis: allograft vs autograft. Orthopedics 1996;19:389–94.
43. Francisco R, Chiodo CP, Wilson MG. Management of the rigid adult acquired flatfoot deformity. Foot Ankle Clin North Am 2007;12:317–27.
44. Knupp M, Stufkens SAS, Hintermann B. Triple arthrodesis. Foot Ankle Clin North Am 2011;16:61–7.
45. Saltzman CL, Fehrle MJ, Cooper RR, et al. Triple arthrodesis: twenty-five and forty-four year average follow-up of the same patients. J Bone Joint Surg Am 1999;81:1391–402.
46. Czurda T, Seidl M, Seiser AS, et al. Triple arthrodesis in treatment of degenerative hindfoot deformities: clinical, radiological and pedobarographic results. Z Orthop Unfall 2009;147:356–61.
47. Child BJ, Hix J, Catanzariti AR, et al. The effect of hindfoot realignment in triple arthrodesis. J Foot Ankle Surg 2009;48:285–93.
48. Jarde O, Abiraad G, Gabrion A, et al. Triple arthrodesis in the management of acquired flatfoot deformity in the adult secondary to posterior tibial tendon dysfunction: a retrospective study of 20 cases. Acta Orthop Belg 2002;68:56–62.
49. Wu WL, Huang PJ, Lin CJ, et al. Lower extremity kinematics and kinetics during level walking and stair climbing in subjects with triple arthrodesis of subtalar fusion. Gait Posture 2005;21:263–70.
50. De Groot IB, Reijman M, Lunig HA, et al. Long-term results after a triple arthrodesis of the hindfoot: function and satisfaction in 36 patients. Int Orthop 2008;32:237–41.
51. Daglar B, Deveci A, Delialioglu OM, et al. Results of triple arthrodesis: effect of primary etiology. J Orthop Sci 2008;13:341–7.
52. Raikin SM. Failure of triple arthrodesis. Foot Ankle Clin 2002;7:121–33.
53. Bono JV, Jacobs RL. Triple arthrodesis through a single lateral approach: a cadaveric experiment. Foot Ankle 1992;13:408–12.

54. Jeng CL, Tankson CJ, Myerson MS. The single medial approach to triple arthrodesis: a cadaver study. Foot Ankle Int 2006;27:1122–5.
55. Jeng CL, Vora AM, Myerson MS. The medial approach to triple arthrodesis. Indications and technique for management of rigid valgus deformities in high-risk patients. Foot Ankle Clin North Am 2005;10:515–21.
56. Inman VT, editor. DuVries' surgery of the foot. 3rd edition. St. Louis: CV Mosby Co.; 1973:491-4.
57. Philippot R, Wegrzyn J, Besse JL. Arthrodesis of the subtalar and talonavicular joints through a medial surgical approach: a series of 15 cases. Arch Orthop Trauma Surg 2010;130:599–603.
58. O'Malley MJ, Deland JT, Lee KT. Selective hindfoot arthrodesis for the treatment of adult acquired flatfoot deformity: an in vitro study. Foot Ankle Int 1995;16:411–7.
59. Astion DJ, Deland JT, Otis JC, et al. Motion of the hindfoot after simulated arthrodesis. J Bone Joint Surg Am 1997;79:241–6.
60. Wülker N, Stukenborg C, Savory KM, et al. Hindfoot motion after isolated and combined arthrodeses: measurements in anatomic specimens. Foot Ankle Int 2000; 21:921–7.
61. Mann RA, Beaman DN. Double arthrodesis in the adult: Clin Orthop Relat Res 1999;365:74–80.
62. Beischer AD, Brodsky JW, Pollo FE, et al. Functional outcome and gait analysis after triple or double arthrodesis. Foot Ankle Int 1999;20:545–53.
63. Thelen S, Rütt J, Wild M, et al. The influence of talonavicular versus double arthrodesis on load dependent motion of the midtarsal joint. Arch Orthop Trauma Surg 2010;130: 47–53.
64. Knupp M, Schuh R, Stufkens SA, et al. Subtalar and talonavicular arthrodesis through a single medial approach for the correction of severe planovalgus deformity. J Bone Joint Surg Br 2009;91:612–5.
65. Brilhault J. Single medial approach to modified double arthrodesis in rigid flatfoot with lateral deficient skin. Foot Ankle Int 2009;30:21–6.
66. Sammarco VJ, Magur EG, Sammarco GJ, et al. Arthrodesis of the subtalar and talonavicular joints for correction of symptomatic hindfoot malalignment. Foot Ankle Int 2006;27:661–6.

Management of the Rigid Arthritic Flatfoot in the Adults
Alternatives to Triple Arthrodesis

Christopher E. Gentchos, MD[a], John G. Anderson, MD[b],*,
Donald R. Bohay, MD[b]

KEYWORDS

- Triple arthrodesis • Flatfoot • Arthritic flatfoot

KEY POINTS

- The goals of the surgical management of the acquired flatfoot deformity are to restore a plantigrade foot that is stable in the stance phase and functional for propulsion.
- Every alternative to triple arthrodesis in the rigid acquired flatfoot deformity is predicated on limiting the patient exposure to the complication associated with triple arthrodesis.
- Successful treatment is dependent on thoughtful patient evaluation and examination, meticulous joint preparation, careful positioning with rigid fixation, and judicious use of adjunctive procedures to achieve the goal of a plantigrade foot that functions well and is minimally painful.

The human foot collapses in a finite number of patterns. This collapse can be driven by injury, time, and weight in a susceptible person. Symptoms occur at various points along the spectrum of the different patterns. But all patterns are united by the common denominator of medial column incompetence and gradual attenuation of the static and dynamic supports of the medial longitudinal and transverse arch in the presence of a progressive triceps surae contracture. Regardless of the cause, it is unclear why the supple deformity becomes rigid. After this threshold has been passed, treatment options become limited to arthrodesis, although there are alternatives to the triple arthrodesis.

Nonarthrodesis surgical solutions to the rigid acquired flatfoot deformity are rarely indicated and rarely performed. To the best of our knowledge, there are no authors or published studies that have recommended joint-sparing procedures for this condition.

The author has nothing to disclose.
[a] Foot & Ankle Orthopaedic Specialist, Concord Orthopaedics PA, 264 Pleasant Street, Concord, NH 03301, USA; [b] Orthopaedic Associates of Michigan, PC, 1111 Leffingwell Avenue, NE, Grand Rapids, MI 49525, USA
* Corresponding author.
E-mail address: John.Anderson@oamichigan.com

Foot Ankle Clin N Am 17 (2012) 323–335
doi:10.1016/j.fcl.2012.03.009
1083-7515/12/$ – see front matter © 2012 Elsevier Inc. All rights reserved.

foot.theclinics.com

However, to contemplate the full breadth of treatment options, particularly adjunctive procedures, surgeons must possess an understanding of the pathogenesis that leads to the deformity and recognize the multiple individual components of that deformity that can be addressed and potentially corrected. Additionally, one must recognize all patterns of collapse to understand the rigid deformity.

The adult acquired flatfoot deformity, in all its various stages of presentation, has become synonymous with dysfunction of the posterior tibial tendon. But this narrow definition of collapse potentially misses other patterns and obscures the common findings in all patterns. The epidemic of obesity that currently plagues our nation has created a unique opportunity. Sufficient numbers of patients are crushing their feet, which allows us to observe an accelerated version of a process that used to take a lifetime to occur.[1] Regardless of the driving force—gravity, time, or a tendency to collapse, the breakdown of the arch in the transverse and sagittal plane is the cornerstone to understanding idiopathic acquired conditions of the foot and ankle and is critical to understanding the treatment of both the supple and the rigid acquired flatfoot deformity correction.

ANATOMY AND PATHOPHYSIOLOGY

Adult flatfoot deformity can result from a developmental cause, including tarsal coalition, congenital vertical talus or neuromuscular conditions,[2] or as an acquired condition in an adult.[1] The principal mechanical contributors to the adult acquired flatfoot are contracture of the triceps surae complex,[3] attenuation of the ligamentous supports of the foot,[1] and posterior tibial tendon (PTT) dysfunction.[4]

The soleus muscle originates on the posterior tibia and the gastrocnemius originates on the posterior distal femur. Depending on the rotation of the hip and the position of the knee, the triceps surae complex has a dynamic effect on the foot, depending on the phase of gait.[1] The Achilles inserts on the posterior tuberosity of the calcaneus, acts though the tibiotalar joint, which sits in the posterior third of the medial longitudinal arch. At mid to late stance, the triceps surae contracts, heel rise and toe off proceed because of a competent medial column and a functional PTT.[4] An incompetent medial column and a dysfunctional posterior tibial tendon prevent full inversion during midstance. This laxity then allows the triceps surae to act through the midfoot instead of the metatarsal heads, leading to further attenuation and collapse. The lack of full excursion of the Achilles then leads to the inevitable tightness, either gastrocnemius or combined Achilles. Not only does gastrocnemius tightness cause symptoms in isolation,[5] but it is ubiquitous in the acquired flatfoot deformity.[6,7]

With the force of the triceps surae acting through the midfoot, ultimately the attenuation progresses across the entire medial column: talonavicular, naviculocuneiform, and tarsometatarsal articulations. The static supports of the arch, plantar fascia, spring ligament, and the talocalcaneal interosseous ligament, also stretch. Finally, compensatory heel valgus ensues due to the progressive forefoot supination. This constellation of progression leads to the radiographic appearance of lateral or dorsilateral peritalar subluxation.[8,9]

The posterior tibial tendon has a normal excursion of only 1.5 to 2.0 cm.[10] As the 5-point attachment of the posterior tibial tendon moves more laterally, the demands on the tendon increase. This accounts for the chronic reparative changes, mucinous degeneration, fibroblast hypercellularity, chondroid metaplasia, and neovascularization[11] that occur in the critical watershed zone: the 14-mm region 1 to 1.5 cm distal to the medial malleolus.[12] A triceps surae contracture is conjectured to contribute to, if not cause, this failure.[7,13] At some point during this process, some threshold is passed and symptoms occur.

An acquired flatfoot deformity is considered rigid when the deformity cannot be passively corrected. There is not universal agreement on this definition since the global deformity involves the hindfoot, transverse tarsal, and midfoot articulations, all of which can have some degree of rigidity. In 1989 Johnson and Strom[14] suggested the simplest definition. A flatfoot is rigid if the hindfoot is stiff and deformed.

There is no logical explanation why some acquired flatfoot deformities become rigid. Ellington and Myerson suggested that the transition from flexible to rigid deformity is a gradual mechanical change during flattening of the arch due to a triceps surae contracture.[15] They further cited 2 other opinions on the cause: habitual overstrain in patients who are developmentally weak[16] and injury to the interosseous ligament of the subtalar joint.[17] The authors opine that progressive capsular contracture is due to chronic joint subluxation in the presence of a triceps surae contracture, medial column incompetence, and progressive muscle imbalance.

CLASSIFICATION

In 1989, Johnson and Strom proposed a classification of posterior tibial tendon dysfunction.[14] This classification was based on the structure and function of the posterior tibial tendon and the position of the foot. The third stage in their classification was defined as an elongated posterior tibial tendon with a fixed hindfoot deformity. Pain is present medially and sometimes laterally and a treatment with arthrodesis was suggested. Myerson[18] expanded this classification to include the acquired flatfoot deformity with the tilted ankle. Several further classifications have also been proposed focusing on the posterior tibial tendon,[19,20] and an algorithmic approach to treatment has also been suggested.[21] Posterior tibial tendon dysfunction stage 3 has also been subdivided into 3A, a deformity that can be corrected by triple arthrodesis, and 3B, with forefoot abduction corrected with additional bone block arthrodesis.[22]

To better guide our understanding and treatment, in 2007, the authors introduced a simple, comprehensive biomechanical model of the distinct types or patterns of foot collapse, including the acquired flatfoot deformity. This model aimed to globally unite idiopathic acquired conditions of the foot and ankle in their relation to medial column incompetence.[23]

Data were collected on 1142 cases, all of which involved at least 1 of 13 different procedure types used for acquired idiopathic foot and ankle conditions. An analysis of these cases showed that there are characteristics common to each of these conditions. These common characteristics, present to varying degrees in idiopathic acquired foot and ankle conditions, were analyzed. Five distinct types or patterns of collapse were identified using data derived from the empirical keying method.[24] These patterns are based on a biomechanical model of progressive medial column incompetence in the presence of a triceps surae contracture and are summarized.

Pattern 1: Precollapse

This pattern involves isolated triceps surae contracture with associated foot pain in the absence of acquired deformity. Foot pain is due to acquired strain in the absence of attenuation of the ligamentous supports of the longitudinal and transverse arch without incompetence of the medial column and without deformity of the talonavicular, naviculocuneiform, intercuneiform, or cuneiform-metatarsal articulations.

Pattern 2: Forefoot

In this pattern, isolated acquired forefoot deformity is the principal component. The ligamentous supports of the foot are attenuated. Forefoot symptoms result from multiplanar instability of the medial column in the presence of a triceps surae contracture, without failure of the transverse arch. Incompetence of the medial column causes greater weight-bearing demands on the more stable second or third ray.

Pattern 3: Midfoot

A clinical flatfoot appearance was present with arch collapse through the midfoot and radiographic evidence of midfoot arthrosis was the principal component. This represents the failure of the transverse arch. Multiple distinct patterns of midtarsal arthrosis exist. In the most common pattern, medial column incompetence in the presence of a triceps surae contracture leads to overload of the more stable second and third rays at the midfoot. The initial point of failure in this type is the more stable second metatarsal–middle cuneiform joint. Medial column incompetence here is suggested as the more stable transverse arch fails by dorsal collapses (dorsal 2nd tarsometatarsal spur). Failure progresses to the third metatarsal–lateral cuneiform joint, followed by the medial navicular–cuneiform articulation, depending on the degree of intercuneiform incompetence.

Pattern 4: Hindfoot

The arch has collapsed. Hindfoot valgus is the principal component. Advanced medial column incompetence in the presence of a triceps surae contracture results in forefoot supination leading to more proximal ligamentous attenuation and compensatory heel valgus, which includes the rigid deformity, and is not limited to cases of symptomatic posterior tibial tendon dysfunction. Radiographic patterns include dorsolateral peritalar subluxation, lateral peritalar subluxation, or overt collapse through the midfoot with hindfoot valgus.

Pattern 5: Ankle

Acquired tilted ankle deformity was the principal component. These patients presented with a clinical flatfoot, hindfoot valgus, and ankle pain or overt arthritis. These ankle deformities were rigid. The triceps surae contracture was advanced, globally involving the gastrocnemius and soleus. In these cases, the acquired flatfoot deformity lead to failure of the final medial restraint, the deltoid ligament, and subsequent ankle valgus.

ALTERNATIVES TO TRIPLE ARTHRODESIS

The goals of the surgical management of the acquired flatfoot deformity are to restore a plantigrade foot that is stable in the stance phase and functional for propulsion. Additionally, since the principal symptom that leads to surgery is pain, a minimally symptomatic foot and ankle should be a principal consideration.

The triple arthrodesis remains a time-tested treatment for the rigid flatfoot deformity, but alternatives exist. Which and how many joints to involve in the arthrodesis remain questions.

Subtalar Arthrodesis

Johnson and Strom favored an isolated subtalar joint arthrodesis over triple arthrodesis to treat the posterior tibial tendon–deficient acquired flatfoot with a deformed and stiff hindfoot.[14] This has been shown to be an effective procedure for stage 2 and 3 deformities[25] as well as when combined with a flexor digitorum longus transfer.[25,26] Indications include less than 30% talonavicular uncovering, isolated symptomatic subtalar joint arthrosis, and isolated lateral foot or sinus pain.[15] Greater than 10° to

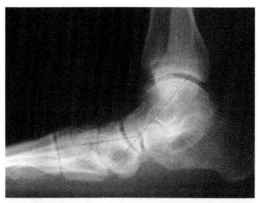

Fig. 1. Preoperative sagittal radiograph of a painful rigid acquired flatfoot deformity. Medial soft tissue was tenuous and isolated subtalar joint arthrodesis was recommended. The forefoot had a fixed 15° varus.

15° of forefoot varus or joint hypermobility is a contraindication to isolated subtalar joint arthrodesis (**Figs. 1–5**).

Mann and colleagues suggested that the fixed forefoot varus could cause excessive load on the lateral border of the foot in this circumstance.[27] In a review of isolated subtalar joint arthrodesis for a host of conditions including congenital and acquired flatfoot deformity (8 of 44), Mann and colleagues[27] reported transverse tarsal motion diminished by 40%, dorsiflexion by 30%, and plantarflexion by 9%. Additionally, they reported a 36% and 41% incidence of mild progression of ankle and transverse tarsal arthritis, respectively. Despite this, the residual motion of the transverse tarsal joints, also reported as 26% and 56% residual mobility, respectively,[28] may diminish the rate of progression of ankle arthrosis when compared to a triple arthrodesis.[29]

The outcomes of isolated subtalar arthrodesis can be good. Kitoaka and Patzer[29] achieved 100% union rate in 21 patients who underwent isolated subtalar joint arthrodesis for treatment of posterior tibial tendon deficient acquired flatfoot, without fixed forefoot varus. The only poor outcome was in one patient who had residual

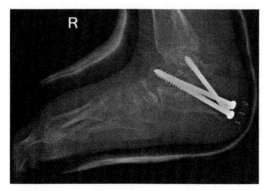

Fig. 2. Immediate postoperative sagittal radiograph shows excellent hindfoot restoration; however, the forefoot remains in a varus position.

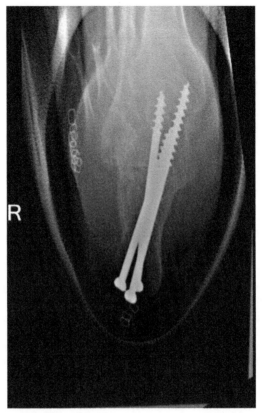

Fig. 3. Immediate postoperative radiographs of an isolated subtalar arthrodesis; an adjunctive tendo-Achilles lengthening was also performed. The axial projection suggested acceptable hindfoot alignment.

hindfoot varus. Deformity was corrected with a 20° increase in talo first metatarsal angle and a 5-mm increase in arch height, both statistically significant.

As expected, overall complication rates are lower for isolated joint arthrodesis, particularly since nonunions more commonly occur at the talonavicular and

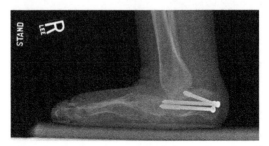

Fig. 4. Lateral standing radiographs show overt failure of the hindfoot alignment and recurrence of the flatfoot deformity 12 months after surgery.

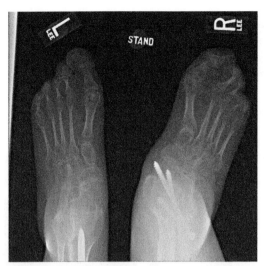

Fig. 5. Anteroposterior radiographs show overt failure of the hindfoot alignment and recurrence of the flatfoot deformity 12 months after surgery.

calcanoecuboid joints with triple arthrodesis.[30] Malunion can also cause a poor result. Mann and colleagues[27] considered the residual motion of the transverse tarsal joint to be protective with an isolated subtalar joint arthrodesis; however, with varus malalignment, the transverse tarsal joint is locked and the compensatory motion is diminished. Easley and colleagues[31] agreed when they reported the results of 184 subtalar joint fusions. There was a 9% incidence of symptomatic varus malunion, 4 of which were considered for hindfoot osteotomy. Careful attention needs to be given to joint position. Hansen[32] demonstrated the use of a lamina spreader carefully placed into the anterior process of the calcaneus and the lateral shoulder of the talus used to open the sinus tarsi and reduce the uncovered talus. This is a powerful tool and overcorrection into varus is possible (**Figs. 6–7**).

Undercorrection, with residual hindfoot valgus, can also lead to progressive midfoot collapse and recalcitrant subfibular impingement.[31] For selected patients with forefoot varus less that 15°, when combined with adjunctive procedures, an isolated subtalar joint arthrodesis can correct the acquired flatfoot deformity with good clinical outcomes.[25]

Surgical Technique

The patient and surgical site are appropriately marked according to hospital or institutional protocol. The procedure is performed under a general anesthetic with a popliteal block. The anticipation is for outpatient surgery, unless compelling reasons mandate an inpatient hospitalization. The patient is positioned supine with thigh tourniquet and an ipsilateral hip bump. Typically the foot retains a considerable external rotational posture despite this and care must be taken to position the leg with the anticipation of deformity correction in mind. Assuming no significant malalignment of the leg exists, the leg is carefully positioned so the knee is directly anterior regardless of the overall resting position of the foot at this stage. Pressure points on the well leg are padded and the patient is secured in position. The authors use the same setup protocol for all procedures reviewed.

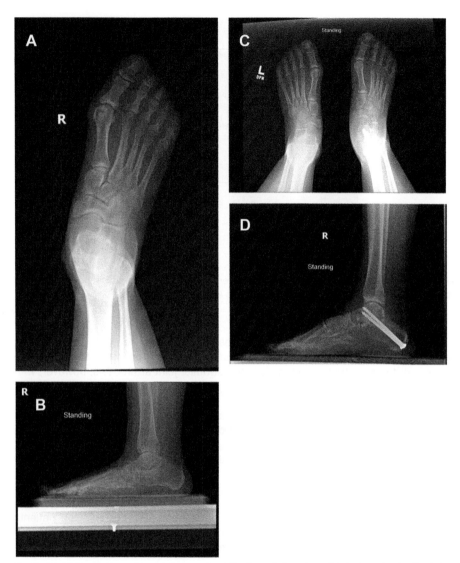

Fig. 6. (A–D) Correction of he rigid acquired flatfoot deformity with isolated subtalar joint arthrodesis, tendo-Achilles lengthening, flexor digitorum longus transfer, and spring liga-ment repair (exostectomy of the talonavicular joint). Lateral hindfoot pain developed 14 months after surgery, likely due to overcorrection of deformity and locking of the transverse tarsal joint.

The authors start with a tendon Achilles lengthening. Typically, a three-incision Hoke procedure is the most effective. The extensile lateral approach is utilized, in line with the fourth metatarsal. The extensor digitorum brevis is elevated. In these deformities, there are typically no remaining soft tissue attachments in the sinus, and the subtalar joint is readily entered. A key elevator is used to primarily disrupt adhesion in the posterior facet. A large lamina spreader is then utilized to progressively distract the joint. Any remaining articular cartilage is then removed

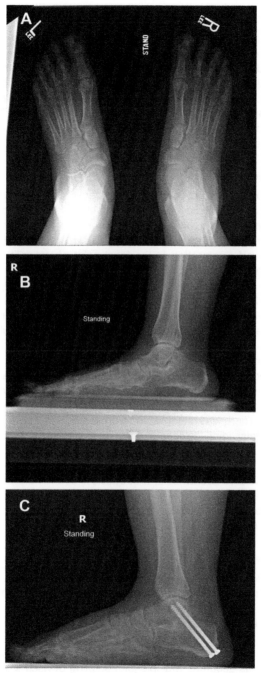

Fig. 7. (*A–C*) Isolated subtalar joint arthrodesis and tendo-Achilles lengthening was preformed restoring sagittal alignment.

until the subchondral bone has been fully denuded. The lamina spreader is repositioned until all articular surfaces have been fully prepared. The exposure is considered adequate and the contracted joint capsule released when the subtalar joint is fully distracted and the flexor hallucis longus tendon can be easily seen in the posterior medial aspect. The joint is irrigated of all loose articular fragments and the subchondral plate is disrupted. The joint is carefully positioned; the lamina spreader technique[32] is the authors preferred method. Once properly positioned the joint is compressed with solid or cannulated lag screws. The authors then proceed to transfer the flexor digitorum longus as well as any further medial column procedures.

Talonavicular Arthrodesis

Isolated talonavicular arthrodesis can be considered in patients with acquired flatfoot deformity who retain some rear foot mobility without evidence of arthrosis in the subtalar joint.[33] An isolated talonavicular arthrodesis cannot correct midtarsal instability or excessive hindfoot valgus,[15] particularly if the hindfoot is stiff. This arthrodesis can provide a powerful correction at the focal point of instability.[34] However, in a cadaver model, while the correction can be the same as a double or triple arthrodesis, hindfoot motion is diminished by 80%.[35] Harper and Tisdel[33,34] reported the results of isolated talonavicular arthrodesis for treatment of adult acquired flatfoot deformity in 26 patients. Their ages ranged from 39 to 74 years, with an average age of 57. The author used a medial approach and fixed the fusion with cannulated screws. He reported the clinical outcome, including any loss of motion, the radiographic results, and the physical appearance of the foot, relative to the contralateral side. The majority of patients retained some hindfoot motion, up to 20°, but was variable. Compared to the contralateral side, ankle loss of motion was 10°, mostly in plantarflexion. The foot was rated as symmetric in appearance in all but 3 patients. Those 3 were assessed as residual valgus. There was radiographic progression of arthrosis in 5 patients. This included the tibiotalar joint, calcaneocuboid joint, and naviculocuneiform joint. An isolated talonavicular arthrodesis can be an effective treatment for the acquired flatfoot deformity. When symptoms are present that can clearly be related to the subtalar joint, an isolated talonavicular arthrodesis is contraindicated. This procedure addresses the apex of the deformity and offers the possibility of a single surgical approach, but does pose the risk of residual hindfoot malalignment. When present, this should be corrected with a hindfoot osteotomy.[36]

Surgical Technique

The authors proceed initially with Hoke tendo-Achilles lengthening. The talonavicular joint is entered through an extensile medial utility incision. The talar head is easily exposed and denuded of articular cartilage. Meticulous preparation of the navicular is typically more challenging and requires frequent repositioning of the lamina spreader to ensure that the subchondral bone is fully exposed. Position needs to be carefully performed but is typically less challenging assuming preoperative assessment of hindfoot mobility was accurate. Multiple joint stapling devises are available, but the authors prefer lag screw fixation. A final screw placed percutaneous on the more lateral aspect of the talonavicular joint can increase the number of lag screws compressing the joint, a possible concern when relying on correction of deformity through the talonavicular joint in isolation. A medializing calcaneus osteotomy can be added if concern exists about foot position.

Double Arthrodesis (Talonavicular and Calcaneocuboid)

The double arthrodesis has been advocated for use in the posterior tibial tendon deficient flatfoot deformity as an alternative to triple arthrodesis.[37,38] Clain and Baxter[37] reported 1 asymptomatic nonunion in 16 patients followed over an 83-month period. Twelve of their patients had a good or excellent result. They reserved this procedure for the rigid flatfoot where the deformity originated in the transverse tarsal joint, and a passively correctable hindfoot valgus. The decision to proceed with a triple arthrodesis was made intraoperative based on the correct-ability of the hindfoot.

Mann and Beaman[38] reviewed the results of 24 double fusions. Their indications were a fixed forefoot varus on 10° to 15° and a subtalar joint that is passively correctable to neutral, with subtalar joint arthrosis as a contraindication. They reported an overall patient satisfaction rate of 83%. Four talonavicular nonunions were reported, and adjacent joint arthrosis was common.

In a review of the rigid adult acquired flatfoot deformity, Francisco and colleagues[39] thought that the constellation of physical findings, the rigid acquired flatfoot with deformity originating at the transverse tarsal joint without significant heel valgus or passively correctable valgus, is uncommon. They reported an alternative double arthrodesis involving the talonavicular and subtalar joints, allowing correction for the hindfoot valgus and forefoot abduction. The authors concur that indications for the double arthrodesis in the rigid acquired flatfoot deformity are rare. Additionally, the functional result of a double arthrodesis in complete loss of hindfoot mobility, we prefer a triple arthrodesis, or a modification as suggested by Francisco and colleagues.[39]

Surgical Technique

The authors initially proceed with Hoke tendo-Achilles lengthening. The talonavicular joint is exposed and prepared as previously described. The lateral hindfoot is then approached through an extensile lateral incision in line with the fourth metatarsal. The calcaneocuboid joint typically is neither difficult to expose nor prepare. Rigid fixation with joint compression is based on surgeon preference.

Adjunctive Procedures

Surgical procedures in addition to arthrodesis should be expected in planning the operative management of the rigid acquired flatfoot deformity. A triceps surae contracture is ubiquitous[6,7] and should be treated with a gastrocnemius recession or tendo-Achilles lengthening. The authors believe that in the more advanced rigid flatfoot deformities, a gastrocnemius lengthening can be inadequate. A tendo-Achilles lengthening is almost always needed and has proved a considerable adjunct to positioning. This is consistent with the suggestion of a progressive triceps surae contracture associated with the more advanced and rigid acquired flatfoot deformities.[15] When considering an isolated subtalar arthrodesis, treating a symptomatic posterior tibial tendon tear with flexor digitorum longus transfer can be critical.[25] Medial column incompetence in the coronal and sagittal plane is also ubiquitous in the acquired flatfoot deformity. Judicious use of medial column stabilization is not readily required in the rigid deformity, particularly since the talonavicular joint is commonly involved in the arthrodesis.

SUMMARY

Every alternative to triple arthrodesis in the rigid acquired flatfoot deformity is predicated on limiting the patient exposure to the complication associated with triple arthrodesis. When possible, avoiding arthrodesis of either the talonavicular and calcaneocuboid joints, with their higher nonunion rates, seems a cogent option. Successful treatment is dependent on thoughtful patient evaluation and examination, meticulous joint preparation, careful positioning with rigid fixation, and judicious use of adjunctive procedures to achieve the goal of a plantigrade foot that functions well and is minimally painful.

REFERENCES

1. Van Boerum DH, Sangeorzan BJ. Biomechanics and pathophysiology of flat foot. Foot Ankle Clin 2003;8(3):419–29.
2. McCormack AP. Ching RP, Sangeorzan BJ. Biomechanics of procedures used in adult flat foot deformity. Foot Ankle Clin 2001;6(1):15–23.
3. Harris, RI, Beath T. Hypermobile flat foot with short tendo Achilles. J Bone Joint Surg Am 1948;30A:116–40.
4. Thordarson DB, Schmotzer H, Chon J, et al. Dynamic support of the human longitudinal arch: a biomechanical evaluation. Clin Orthop 1995;316:165–72.
5. Digiovanni CW, Kuo R, Tejwani N, et al. Isolated gastrocnemius tightness. J Bone Joint Surg 2002;84:962–70.
6. Coetzee JC, Castro MD. The indications and biomechanical rationale for various hindfoot procedures in the treatment of posterior tibialis tendon dysfunction. Foot Ankle Clin 2003;8:453–9.
7. DiGiovanni CW, Langer P. The role of isolated gastrocnemius and combined Achilles contractures in the flatfoot. Foot Ankle Clin 2007;12:363–79.
8. Anderson JG, Hansen ST. Surgical treatment of posterior tendon pathology. In Kelikien AS, editor. Operative treatment of the foot and ankle. Stanford (CT): Appleton & Lange; 1999. p. 211–3.
9. Hansen ST. Functional reconstruction of the foot and ankle. Baltimore (MD): Williams & Wilkins; 2000: p. 195–207.
10. Mann RA. Biomechanics of the foot and ankle. In Mann RA, Coughlin MJ, editors. Surgery of the foot and ankle. St Louis (MO): Mosby; 1993. p. 3–43.
11. Mosier SM, Lucas DR. Pomeroy GC, et al. Pathology of the posterior tibial tendon in posterior tibial tendon insufficiency. Foot Ankle Int 1998;19:520–4.
12. Frey CC, Schereff M, Greenidge N. Vascularity of the posterior tibial tendon. J Bone Joint Surg Am 1990;72: 884–8.
13. Mosier SM, Pomeroy G, Manoli A. Pathoanatomy and etiology of posterior tibial tendon dysfunction. Clin Orthop 1999;365:12–22.
14. Johnson KA, Strom DE. Tibialis posterior tendon dysfunction. Clin Orthop 1989;239: 196–206.
15. Ellington JK, Myerson MS. The use of arthrodesis to correct rigid flatfoot deformity. Instruc Course Lec 2011;60:311–20.
16. Todd AH. The treatment of pes cavus. Proc R Soc Med 1934;28(2):117–28.
17. Lapidus PW. The so-called longitudinal arch: some new thoughts. Am J Phys Anthropol 1948;6(2):241.
18. Myerson MS. Adult acquired flatfoot deformity: treatment of dysfunction of the posterior tibial tendon. J Bone Joint Surg 1996;78:780–92.
19. Conti S, Michelson J, Jahss M. Clinical significance of magnetic resonance imaging in preoperative planning for reconstruction of posterior tibial tendon ruptures. Foot Ankle 1992;13:208–14.
20. Cooper AJ, Mizel MS, Patel PD, et al. Comparison of MRI and local anesthetic tendon sheath injection in the diagnosis of posterior tibial tendon tenosynovitis. Foot Ankle Int 2007;28:1124–7.

21. Weinraub GM, Heilala MA. Adult flat foot/posterior tibial tendon dysfunction; outcomes analysis of surgical treatment utilizing an algorithmic approach. J Foot Ankle Surg 2000;39:359–64.
22. Bluman EC, Title CI, Myerson MS. Posterior tibial tendon rupture: a refined classification. Foot Ankle Clin 2007;12:233–49.
23. Gentchos CE, Jelenick A, Bohay DR, et al. Patterns of arch collapse associated with progressive gastrocnemius contracture. Presented at the annual scientific meeting of the American Orthopaedic Foot and Ankle Society. Toronto (Canada), July 2007.
24. Hathaway SR, McKinley JC. Minnesota Multiphasic Personality Inventory revised. Minneapolis (MN): University of Minnesota Press; 1943.
25. Johnson JE, Cohen BE, DiGiovanni BF, et al. Subtalar arthrodesis with flexor digitorum longus transfer and spring ligament repair for treatment of posterior tibial tendon insufficiency. Foot Ankle Int 2000;21(9):722–9.
26. Stephens HM, Walling AK, Solmen JD, et al. Subtalar repositional arthrodesis for adult acquired flatfoot. Clin Orthop Rel Res 1999;365:69–73.
27. Mann RA, Beaman, DM, Horton GA. Isolated subtalar arthrodesis. Foot Ankle Int 1998;19(8):511–9.
28. Astion DJ, Deland JT, Otis JC, et al. Motion of the hindfoot after simulated arthrodesis. J Bone Joint Surg Am 1997;79:241–6.
29. Kitaoka HB, Patzer GL. Subtalar arthrodesis for posterior tibial tendon dysfunction and pes planus. Clin Orthop Rel Res 1997;345:187–94.
30. Kadakia AR, Haddad SL. Hindfoot arthrodesis for the adult acquired flat foot. Foot Ankle Clin 2003;8(3):569–94.
31. Easley ME, Trnka HJ, Schon LC, et al. Isolated subtalar joint arthrodesis. J Bone Joint Surg Am 2000;82(A):613–24.
32. Hansen ST. Functional reconstruction of the foot and ankle. Baltimore (MD): Williams & Wilkins; 2000. p. 302–3.
33. Harper MC, Tisdel CL. Talonavicular arthrodesis for the painful adult acquired flatfoot deformity. Foot Ankle Int 1996;17(11):658–61.
34. Harper MC. Talonavicular arthrodesis for the acquired flatfoot in adults. Clin Orthop Relat Res 1999;365:65–8.
35. O'MalleyMJ, Deland JT, Lee KT. Selective hindfoot arthrodesis for the treatment of acquired flatfoot deformity: an in vitro study. Foot Ankle Int 1995;16(7):411–7.
36. Fortin PT. Posterior tibial tendon insufficiency. Isolated fusion of the talonavicular joint. Foot Ankle Clin 2001;6(1):137–51.
37. Clain MR, Baxter DE. Simultaneous calcaeocuboid and talonavicular fusion. Long term follow up study. J Bone Joint Surg Br 1994;76(1):133–6.
38. Mann RA, Beaman DN. Double arthrodesis in the adult. Clin Orthop Rel Res 1999; 365:74–80.
39. Francisco R, Chiodo CP, Wilson MG. Management of the rigid adult acquired flatfoot deformity. Foot Ankle Clin 2007;12:317–27.

Minimizing the Role of Fusion in the Rigid Flatfoot

Ross Taylor, MD[a],*, V. James Sammarco, MD,[b]

KEYWORDS

• Flatfoot • Fusion alternatives • Osteotomy • Reconstruction

KEY POINTS

• Equinus contracture, ankle and hindfoot valgus, midfoot abduction, and forefoot varus must each be individually considered with the ultimate goal of not only deformity correction, but preservation of function in the ankle, subtalar, hindfoot, or midfoot joints.

• Although triple arthrodesis affords predictable correction and pain relief, the long-term sequelae of extended hindfoot fusions include arthritis and often the need for further, more extensive fusion procedures.

• Satisfactory results can be achieved in the rigid flatfoot by limiting fusion to joints that are arthritic, and correcting associated deformity with osteotomy and soft tissue reconstruction.

There has been a proliferation of treatment options for flexible flatfoot deformity, but in cases where the deformities are more rigid and fixed, triple arthrodesis remained the most common surgical technique employed for treatment. Although triple arthrodesis can afford excellent deformity correction, it can be associated with disability owing to the stiffness created by the procedure. Patients may complain of continued pain with ambulation and extended weight bearing or when walking long distances. In addition, after triple arthrodesis, symptomatic arthritis often develops with time in the ankle, midfoot, and intertarsal joints. Extending the arthrodesis when progressive arthritis develops rarely improves the patient's function to their expectation. Converting a triple arthrodesis to a pan-talar arthrodesis leads to a very stiff and often chronically painful leg and, in the authors' opinion, should be avoided. Recognizing both the early and late problems associated with extended hindfoot fusions, increased interest in using the techniques developed for correction of flexible flatfoot has occurred. This dialogue

[a] Coastal Orthopedics, 2376 Cypress Circle Suite 300, Conway, SC 29526, USA; [b] Cincinnati Sports Medicine & Orthopaedic Center, 10663 Montgomery Road, Cincinnati, OH, USA
* Corresponding author.
E-mail address: rtaylor897@sc.rr.com

Foot Ankle Clin N Am 17 (2012) 337–349
http://dx.doi.org/10.1016/j.fcl.2012.03.010
1083-7515/12/$ – see front matter © 2012 Elsevier Inc. All rights reserved.

is intended to provide alternatives to fusion surgery for the treatment of rigid flatfoot deformity while discussing the various osteotomy and soft tissue reconstructive options that may allow the surgeon to either avoid fusion or perform a more limited fusion than might otherwise be required.

DEFORMITY AND ARTHRITIS

Deformity correction without arthrodesis requires a conceptual change for most surgeons, and for patients as well. As a surgeon, one wants to offer the patient a reliable way to fix the problem at hand. In both the rigid and flexible flatfoot, arthrodesis is undoubtedly the most predictable way to achieve a plantigrade foot. When done correctly, there is little chance of deformity recurrence, and pain relief is typically good. The longer term problems associated with arthrodesis can be easily overlooked, but need to be balanced with the need for successful treatment today. This balance needs to be explained to the patient, who must be aware that surgery in the future may be inevitable whether the triple arthrodesis is done primarily or whether arthrodesis is deferred to a later time in life when the patient is not as active. Further individualization of the procedure needs to be done based on the patient's age, activity level, and medical comorbidities.

As the treatment paradigm shifts from fusion to osteotomy, the surgeon must distinguish between components of the flatfoot deformity that are arthritic versus those that are supple and nonarthritic. Once determined, the surgeon may restrict fusion only to those joints that are arthritic while correcting nonarthritic components of the deformity by osteotomy and soft-tissue reconstruction. Equinus contracture, ankle and hindfoot valgus, midfoot abduction, and forefoot varus must each be individually considered with the ultimate goal of not only deformity correction, but preservation of function in the ankle, subtalar, hindfoot, or midfoot joints.

Ankle deformity must be defined before any surgery done to correct flatfoot. Coronal plane valgus deformity of the mortise need to be addressed and may require osteotomy of the tibia to correct bony malalignment, or possibly reconstruction of the attenuated deltoid ligament complex when the talus is tilted in a neutral mortise. Almost all flatfoot correction is associated with equinus owing to posterior muscular contracture, and this is addressed by muscular or tendinous lengthening. Subtalar joint valgus may be rigid even in the absence of arthritis. Conditions such as tarsal coalition or other congenital deformities of the calcaneus may be present with little arthritis of the subtalar joint and may be salvageable without fusion by resection, osteotomy, or both (**Fig. 1**). The traverse tarsal joint is comprised of the talonavicular and calcaneocuboid joints, and deformity here is usually defined by collapse of the arch in the sagittal plane and abduction of the foot through the joint in the axial plane. Correction of both sagittal and axial deformities of the talonavicular joint may be possible by spring ligament reconstruction and digital flexor tendon transfer to the navicular. Further correction can be achieved by lengthening the lateral column through an osteotomy in the calcaneus. Fixed varus deformity in the medial column can be corrected by plantar flexion osteotomy of the medial column. In this way, each deformity segment can be defined, and the surgeon can use what tools are available for correction of the deformity. In the foot, if arthritis of a joint is present, fusion is usually recommended at that segment. When ankle arthritis as present, it is increasingly possible for the surgeon to correct the underlying foot deformity, and perform a staged ankle replacement.

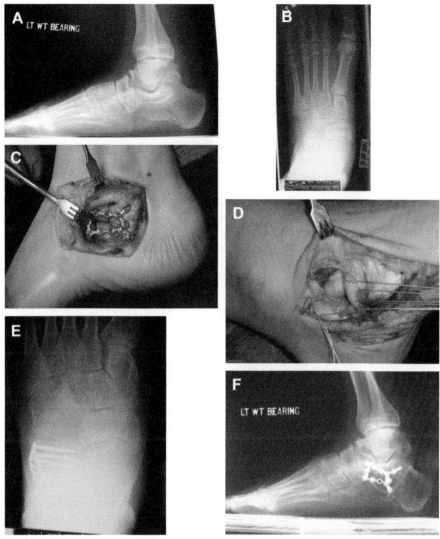

Fig. 1. (*A, B*) A 15-year-old boy with rigid pes planovalgus owing to a middle facet talar-calcaneal coalition. (*C, D*) Surgery included resection of the coalition, MDCO, lateral column lengthening, and advancement of the posterior tibial tendon and reefing of the spring ligament complex. (*E, F*) The patient underwent bilateral procedures and was able to return to high school athletics. X-rays 4 years after procedure demonstrate durable correction without progression of arthritis.

MINIMIZING FUSION: THE ROLE OF OSTEOTOMY AND SOFT-TISSUE RECONSTRUCTION

The contributions of equinus contracture, ankle and hindfoot valgus, midfoot abduction, and forefoot varus in rigid flatfoot deformity are presented. Although many of these deformities have historically been treated with fusion, osteotomy, and soft-tissue reconstructive options for each of these elements of the rigid planovalgus foot are reviewed.

Equinus Contracture

Harris and Beath[1] were the first to identify the role of equinus contracture in flatfoot deformity. With the hindfoot pathologically everted, the Achilles tendon insertion is not only lateralized, but the triceps surae is relatively shortened. Clinical examination may paradoxically suggest a relative increase in dorsiflexion as the foot subluxes laterally and dorsally around the talus with dorsally directed forefoot pressure. Often, it is only with manual reduction of hindfoot valgus that deficits in ankle dorsiflexion become apparent. Rigid hindfoot deformity precludes clinical assessment of equinus contracture until the subtalar joint is reduced at the time of fusion surgery. Numerous authors have supported either tendo-Achilles lengthening (TAL) or gastrocnemius recession as a component of hindfoot reconstruction.[2,3] Lengthening of the triceps surae is, therefore, nearly universally employed by the authors as a component of flatfoot reconstruction both with and without arthrodesis of the subtalar joint. Although there is little controversy regarding the need for this procedure to obtain adequate deformity correction there are 2 differing approaches: Gastrocnemius recession and TAL.

The decision to perform either gastrocnemius recession or TAL at the time of surgical reconstruction of the rigid flatfoot classically depends on the ability to neutralize equinus contracture by flexing the knee (Silfverskiold test).[4] Knee flexion relaxes the gastrocnemius, but not the soleus; the former originates proximal to the knee and the latter distally. An equinus contracture eliminated by knee flexion indicates an isolated gastrocnemius contracture. Conversely, persistence of equinus contracture with knee flexion indicates contracture of the entire triceps surae or a shortened Achilles tendon. Although TAL lengthens the entire triceps surae group, gastrocnemius recession provides selective lengthening of the superficial muscles only. Proponents of TAL cite its simplicity, ease, and cosmesis versus a gastrocnemius recession. Unfortunately, TAL has been associated with tendon rupture.[5] It is our experience that overlengthening of the tendon with loss of push-off is common with TAL in adults, and that the incised Achilles tendon can be a source of persistent pain. Although gastrocnemius recession has been shown to provide predictable correction of equinus deformity,[6] risks include sural nerve injury and unacceptable cosmesis.

Ankle Valgus

One of the major goals in treatment of flatfoot deformity is the restoration of coronal plane alignment to the ankle and foot. Coronal plane malalignment may occur either as a result of valgus angulation of the tibial plafond secondary to congenital tibial deformity or trauma, or as a result of valgus tilt of the talus due to progression of deltoid ligament insufficiency. As is the case with hindfoot deformity, ankle valgus may be either flexible or rigid. This distinction is reflected in Myerson's expanded the classification of posterior tendon insufficiency to include stage IV. Stage IV-A describes reducible ankle valgus whereas stage IV-B describes rigid ankle valgus.[7]

Traditionally, arthrodesis of the ankle was used to correct significant coronal or sagittal plane malalignment. Although deformity correction is assured and the risk of recurrence is eliminated with this approach, the long-term effects of arthrodesis of the ankle are concerning, particularly where foot deformity requires additional fusion for correction. Progressive arthritis of the peritalar joints after ankle arthrodesis may lead to the eventual need for pantalar arthrodesis, a risk that may be compounded by preexisting flatfoot deformity. We therefore recommend that in cases of significant pes planovalgus, all attempts at preserving the ankle with a joint-sparing procedure be made. With the advent of more successful ankle replacement designs, our philosophy has changed from one where the patient is simply braced until fusion is necessary to one where alignment and ligamentous stability are surgically restored in preparation for a staged joint replacement. With this being said, it is impressive how many patients have significant improvement in their symptoms with deformity correction and restoration of stability despite radiographically significant arthritis of the ankle.

In cases where the distal tibial plafond has a significant valgus deformity, osteotomy of the tibia needs to be considered as part of the reconstruction. There are many techniques to accomplish this including those that use direct realignment by opening or closing wedge osteotomy, and those that favor progressive correction with an external fixator. In cases where valgus exists owing to fracture malunion, deformity correction is straightforward and often can be accomplished by osteotomy of the tibia at the level of the deformity (**Fig. 2**). Congenital cases or cases owing to growth plate disturbance can be more complex as the deformity may be multiplanar. Computed tomography can be particularly helpful in planning these osteotomies and helps to define the amount of valgus and plantar flexion requiring correction. We prefer a closing wedge osteotomy when reconstructing congenital deformity in adults because metaphyseal osteotomies in this area heal quickly with bone on bone apposition, and the slight shortening of the limb that occurs with removal of a wedge of bone decreases soft tissue tension and promotes postoperative motion. The distal tibial articular angle should be corrected to 3% to 5% of valgus, although a neutral angle is acceptable. It is important to avoid overcorrection with varus angulation of the tibial plafond as this may result in unacceptable lateral ankle instability or lateral column overload of the foot. In cases where significant arthritis is present, or in cases where rigid equinus accompanies the deformity, an anterior closing wedge osteotomy can be incorporated to restore neutral sagittal plane alignment of the ankle.

Patients with a normal distal tibial articular angle and reducible valgus tilting of the talus within the ankle mortis (stage IV-A deformity) may be candidates for joint sparing reconstruction. Jeng and colleagues[8] outlined criteria for joint sparing reconstruction as:

- Persistent ankle pain refractory to conservative care;
- Rigid hindfoot valgus and forefoot abduction consistent with stage IV adult acquired flatfoot deformity;
- Valgus tilting of the talus within the mortise of at least 3° that is passively correctible under fluoroscopy; and
- No less than 2 mm of lateral tibiotalar cartilage remaining as measured on standing anteroposterior ankle radiographs.

Joint-sparing procedures involve deltoid ligament reconstruction combined with distal realignment. Although numerous joint-sparing procedures have been described, they uniformly involve reconstruction of the incompetent deltoid ligament. Although procedures involving repair and advancement of the native deltoid ligament have been described, these rely on the repair of diseased tissue and may be predisposed to failure. Reconstruction of the deltoid ligament has been described using both host and native tissues. Deland and associates[9] performed deltoid ligament reconstruction using peroneus longus autograft transferred through bone tunnels to recreate both the superficial and deep components of the deltoid ligament. Jeng and colleagues[8] recently described minimally invasive deltoid ligament reconstruction in combination with triple arthrodesis. Successful outcomes occurred in 5 of 8 patients, underscoring the challenging nature of this condition and the limitations of surgical reconstruction. Most recently, Haddad and colleagues[10] described reconstruction of the superficial and deep deltoid ligaments using tibialis anterior tendon

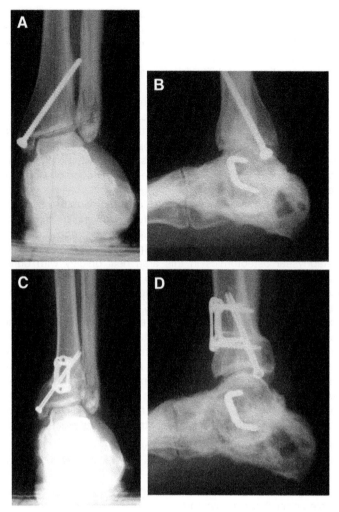

Fig. 2. (*A, B*) Preoperative x-rays of a 32-year-old woman who underwent previous surgery for trauma at age 17 for an open ankle fracture. Note the deficiency of the fibula. She in the intervening years she had undergone several procedures, including triple arthrodesis. She presented with equinus and valgus. X-rays and physical examination revealed that the deformity was at the ankle. (*C, D*) Postoperative films showing anterior and medial biplanar closing wedge osteotomy. Despite radiographic arthritis, the patient experienced dramatic improvement in symptoms.

allograft in 6 cadaveric specimens. Torque testing of reconstructed specimens revealed equivalent resistance to eversion and external rotation to matched controls. Although the initial study was cadaveric, this technique has been performed in eight patients using semitendonosis allograft.

Whereas the goal of restoration of ankle alignment is long-term preservation of ankle function, often arthritis of the ankle progresses despite successful deformity correction. Nonetheless, a well-aligned ankle not only improves overall gait mechanics, but may delay the onset of arthritic symptoms as well. Ultimately, conversion to ankle replacement or even fusion is greatly facilitated by the normal ankle alignment imparted by either osteotomy or deltoid ligament reconstruction.

Hindfoot Valgus

Medial displacement calcaneal osteotomy (MDCO) has been used as an adjunctive procedure in the correction of flexible flatfoot for more than a century. Gleich in 1893 described medializing osteotomy of the calcaneus by excising a medial wedge. Almost a century later in 1960, Dwyer[11] introduced a lateral closing wedge osteotomy of the calcaneus in the treatment of pes cavus deformity. Koutsogiannis[12] in 1971 introduced the idea of a pure medial translational osteotomy of the calcaneus for flatfoot deformity. Since that time, MDCO has gained near universal acceptance as a fundamental component of flexible flatfoot reconstruction. Although studies specifically addressing the use of MDCO in the treatment of rigid flatfoot are lacking, biomechanical principles support its application when combined with both soft-tissue reconstruction and hindfoot fusion.

Coronal plane alignment of the foot is typically restored at the time of hindfoot fusion via internal rotation of calcaneus beneath the talus and with simultaneous reduction of the talonavicular joint. Nonetheless, the degree of obtainable reduction by this method is limited. Although the amount of acceptable hindfoot valgus after subtalar arthrodesis has never been precisely quantified, persistent eversion of the heel has been correlated with ankle degeneration after malaligned hindfoot fusion. Valgus tibiotalar arthritis was observed after valgus malunion of 6 hindfoot fusions in a series of patients reviewed by Fitzgibbons.[13] Furthermore, after hindfoot fusion, preexisting deltoid ligament attenuation as well as posterior tibial tendon insufficiency may act synergistically with residual hindfoot valgus to accelerate postoperative ankle deformity and arthritis. Resnick and colleagues[14] noted a 76% increase in deltoid ligament strain with a valgus displaced hindfoot in a cadaveric triple arthrodesis model. Others have noted marked progression of ankle osteoarthritis after triple arthrodesis.[15,16] It is plausible to assume that residual hindfoot valgus may play a role in deltoid ligament failure and progression to valgus arthritis of the ankle after triple arthrodesis. Medialization of the posterior tuberosity of the calcaneus translates the limb center of gravity toward the medial malleolus, which not only reduces lateral tibiotalar contact forces, but also decreases deltoid ligament strain.

Complete reduction of hindfoot valgus at the time of surgery is necessary for rigid flatfoot deformity, whether surgery includes a subtalar arthrodesis or not. In cases of subtalar arthrodesis, MDCO should be done if residual hindfoot valgus is greater than 7° after provisional fixation. When hindfoot reconstruction is combined with deltoid ligament reconstruction for stage IV deformity, correction of the calcaneus to neutral or 0° is desirable. Inclusion of MDCO as a component of either soft-tissue reconstruction or fusion surgery for the rigid flatfoot may protect the ankle joint from subsequent valgus deformity and degenerative arthritis, ultimately mitigating the risk of requiring ankle fusion.

Midfoot Abduction

In the acquired flatfoot, dorsolateral peritalar subluxation of the tarsus occurs as the posterior tibial tendon and spring ligament fail resulting in midfoot abduction and hindfoot valgus. Evans[17] first demonstrated in the pediatric flatfoot that lateral column lengthening through the anterior body of the calcaneus improved not only midfoot abduction but hindfoot valgus as well. Sangeorzan and colleagues[18] applied lateral column lengthening to the correction of adult acquired flatfoot. In 2003, Anderson subclassified Johnson and Strom stage II into subtypes A and B to quantify the degree of lateral navicular peritalar subluxation as measured on standing AP radiographs.[19] Subgroup B represents patients with greater than 50% uncovering of the talar head and those whom require lateral column lengthening for correction of midfoot abduction.

Much of the controversy surrounding this procedure centers on whether to lengthen the lateral column of the foot with osteotomy of the calcaneus or by distraction arthrodesis of the calcaneocuboid joint. Proponents of the former cite the risk of calcaneocuboid arthritis after lateral column calcaneal lengthening. Cooper and colleagues[20] used a cadaveric model to demonstrate an 8-fold increase in calcaneocuboid joint pressure after lateral column calcaneal lengthening. Proponents of osteotomy cite the potential drawbacks of arthrodesis including not only the diminished hindfoot motion but risk of nonunion as well. Deland and colleagues[21] demonstrated a 52% reduction in talonavicular motion and a 30% reduction in subtalar motion after distraction arthrodesis of the calcaneocuboid joint. Toolan and colleagues[22] reported a 20% rate of nonunion in their series of 41 feet undergoing distraction arthrodesis of the calcaneocuboid joint combined with medial column fusions and FDL transfer. In addition to nonunion, lateral pain owing to overcorrection is more common with distraction arthrodesis of the calcaneocuboid joint than with lateral column calcaneal lengthening; therefore, we reserve distraction arthrodesis of the calcaneocuboid joint for cases where significant arthritis of that joint is present.

Forefoot Varus

Hindfoot valgus and midfoot abduction require compensatory supination of the forefoot to maintain floor contact while standing. Initially flexible, forefoot supination with time may become rigid, resulting in fixed forefoot varus. Malalignment, instability, and arthritis may occur through the talonavicular, naviculocuneiform, or first tarso-metatarsal joints. Whether forefoot varus is a primary or secondary deformity in acquired flatfoot deformity is of ongoing debate. There is, however, little controversy that failure to address fixed forefoot varus at the time of flatfoot reconstruction may result in a supinated forefoot, lateral column overload, and even fracture of the fifth metatarsal.

The distinction between rigid and flexible forefoot varus is important in determining the scope of flatfoot reconstruction. Flexible deformity seldom requires correction unless medial column instability is present on lateral radiographs. The flexibility of forefoot varus is easily evaluated preoperatively when hindfoot deformity is supple. Simultaneous reduction of heel eversion while the ankle is plantar flexed should reduce the forefoot to neutral with minimal coaxing if forefoot varus is flexible. Fixed forefoot varus is more difficult to detect when hindfoot deformity is rigid, because hindfoot reduction may not be possible until correction is done at the time of surgery. Because correction of coronal plane alignment in the flatfoot requires inversion of the subtalar joint, hindfoot correction may exacerbate forefoot varus, particularly when combined with lateral column lengthening. This can be compensated for to a certain extent by increasing plantarflexion of the medial column at the talonavicular joint if arthrodesis of that joint is planned. If the talonavicular joint can be spared, however, forefoot varus can be corrected by medial column osteotomy.

Cotton[23] first described the utility of plantar flexion osteotomy of the medial cuneiform in correcting depression of the medial arch in pes planus. Since then, this osteotomy has been readily adapted to the reconstruction of congenital flatfoot. Hirose and Johnson[24] combined the Cotton osteotomy with hindfoot reconstruction in 16 feet with flatfoot deformity, reporting improved radiographic parameters including lateral talo-first metatarsal angle, calcaneal pitch and medial cuneiform height. Benthien and colleagues[25] demonstrated not only correction of forefoot varus but also diminished lateral column overload after lateral column lengthening with the addition of opening wedge osteotomy of the medial cuneiform in a severe flatfoot model. Unless gross instability or arthritis of the naviculocuneiform or tarsometatarsal joints is present, the authors utilize plantar flexion osteotomy of the medial cuneiform to correct rigid forefoot varus rather than an extended medial column arthrodesis.

LIMITED HINDFOOT FUSIONS

Osteotomy and soft tissue reconstruction can provide surprisingly good correction of even rigid planovalgus deformity; however, the presence of arthritic changes of the subtalar or transverse tarsal joint are a contraindication to this type of joint sparing reconstruction. Triple arthrodesis remains the procedure of choice when long-standing deformity has progressed to severe arthritis, although this procedure is not without its own complications. Most notably, the reported progression of arthritis at the ankle joint after triple arthrodesis has been alarming. Wetmore and Drennan[15] reported a radiographic prevalence of ankle arthritis of 77% and a clinical prevalence of 63% after triple arthrodesis. Pell and colleagues[16] examined 132 feet after triple arthrodesis and noted radiographic progression of ankle osteoarthritis in 60% of their study population. Other studies have demonstrated significant complications including infection, nonunion, malunion, and hardware related problems. Although triple arthrodesis may be the only appropriate surgical procedure in some patients with rigid flatfoot, more limited fusions, including isolated subtalar arthrodesis and double arthrodesis of the subtalar and talonavicular joints, may be reasonable alternatives, particularly when all associated deformities are corrected with soft-tissue reconstruction and osteotomy.

Patients with rigid flatfoot deformities who have a rigid hindfoot valgus deformity yet retain flexibility at the transverse tarsal joint are well-suited for isolated subtalar arthrodesis. Some examples include posttraumatic deformity owing to fracture of the os calcis and rigid pes planovalgus associated with tarsal coalition of the subtalar joint. Mann and colleagues[26] described 5 patients in a larger series of 48 feet who underwent isolated subtalar arthrodesis for posterior tibial tendon dysfunction. The authors noted that "subtalar arthrodesis is indicated in the older, less-active patient when the primary deformity is hindfoot valgus and/or subtalar inversion is absent. If forefoot varus of greater than 10 to 15° or transverse tarsal joint hyper-mobility is present, a subtalar fusion is contraindicated, and a double or triple arthrodesis is indicated."[26] It has been our experience that if the transverse tarsal joint is nonarthritic, it may be possible to correct the forefoot abduction by spring ligament repair and plantar flexion osteotomy of the medial cuneiform. The addition of a flexor digitorum longus transfer to subtalar arthrodesis has been advocated not only for treatment of the flexible flatfoot, but may improve both deformity and function in patients requiring subtalar arthrodesis for rigid deformity.[26] Spring ligament reconstruction also can correct sagittal and axial abduction in these patients if arthritis is absent. Although this patient population may be limited, those with acquired pes planus who retain a supple midfoot in the setting of isolated subtalar arthritis may benefit from isolated subtalar versus triple arthrodesis.

For the patient with arthritis of the subtalar and talonavicular joints, a more extensive arthrodesis is indicated. Traditionally, these patients have undergone a triple arthrodesis, which includes the calcaneocuboid joint into the fusion mass regardless of the presence or absence of calcaneocuboid arthritis. Surgeons have argued that fusion of the calcaneocuboid joint is necessary to achieve adequate

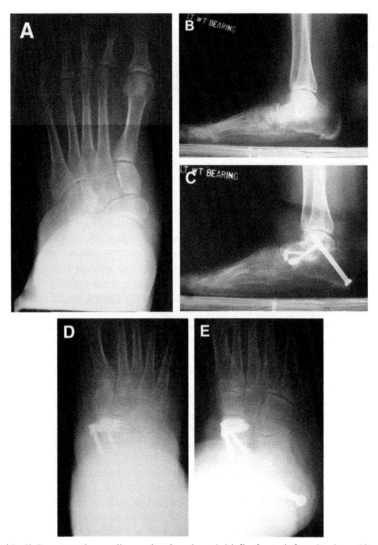

Fig. 3. (*A, B*) Preoperative radiographs showing rigid flatfoot deformity in a 48-year-old woman with disabling pain. Intraoperatively, the subtalar and talonavicular joints were noted to be arthritic, but the calcaneocuboid joint had normal articular cartilage. (*C–E*) Postoperative radiographs demonstrating excellent correction with double arthrodesis and preservation of the calcaneocuboid joint.

deformity correction and to improve the likelihood of successful arthrodesis of the talonavicular joint. The absence of calcaneocuboid joint motion after subtalar and talonavicular joint fusion has been supported by biomechanical studies.[27] Still, these studies do not account for smaller motion, which can help to dissipate force across the lateral column of the foot. It has been these authors' experience that, despite successful realignment with triple arthrodesis, some patients continue to experience pain and discomfort along the lateral aspect of the foot. Preserving the nonarthritic calcaneocuboid joint diminishes this problem. Although reported nonunion rates after

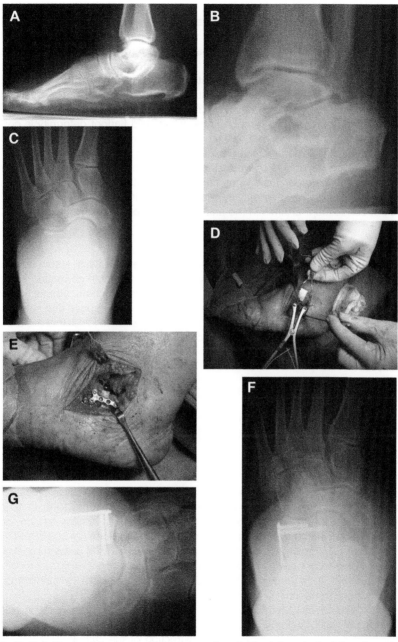

Fig. 4. (*A–C*) A 62-year-old woman with symptomatic arthritis of the subtalar joint after calcaneal fracture. Rigid pes planovalgus was present despite the absence of arthritis in the TN and CC joints. (*D, E*) Subtalar arthrodesis was combined with lateral column lengthening and FDL transfer to spare the transverse tarsal joint. Iliac crest allograft was secured with a locking plate. (*F, G*) Two-year postoperative radiographs showing correction of deformity and successful arthrodesis of the subtalar joint without progression of arthritis at the transverse tarsal joint.

modern triple arthrodesis are low, nonunion not uncommonly involves the calcaneocuboid joint[16,28]; hence, excluding the calcaneocuboid joint from the fusion eliminates the risk of symptomatic calcaneocuboid nonunion. Furthermore, a relative lateral column lengthening is created via talonavicular arthrodesis and calcaneocuboid preservation, directly improving midfoot abduction. Sammarco and colleagues[2] described not only good deformity correction, but also improved function and high rates of patient satisfaction with isolated subtalar and talonavicular arthrodesis in 15 patients with rigid flatfoot deformity (**Fig. 3**).

Although hindfoot fusion is often required when rigid flatfoot deformity is complicated by arthritis, the authors routinely employ osteotomy and soft-tissue reconstruction to correct ankle deformity, hindfoot valgus, midfoot abduction, and forefoot varus while confining fusion only to the subtalar and/or the talonavicular joint if necessary. Judicious use of hindfoot fusion combined with nonfusion reconstructive options offers the patient not only deformity correction, but optimizes function while reducing the risk of subsequent arthritis in the ankle and midfoot joints (**Fig. 4**).

SUMMARY

The goals of surgery for the rigid flatfoot are to achieve a painless, stable, functional plantigrade foot. Although triple arthrodesis affords predictable correction and pain relief, the long-term sequelae of extended hindfoot fusions include arthritis and often the need for further, more extensive fusion procedures. We propose that satisfactory results can be achieved in the rigid flatfoot by limiting fusion to joints that are arthritic, and correcting associated deformity with osteotomy and soft tissue reconstruction.

REFERENCES

1. Harris RI, Beath T. Hypermobile flat-foot with short tendo Achilles. J Bone Joint Surg Am 1948;30:116–41.
2. Sammarco VJ, Magur EG, Sammarco GJ, et al. Arthrodesis of the subtalar and talonavicular joints for correction of symptomatic hindfoot malalignment. Foot Ankle Int 2006;27:661–6.
3. Kadakia AR, Haddad SL. Hindfoot arthrodesis for the adult acquired flatfoot. Foot Ankle Clin 2003;8:569–94.
4. Silver CM, Simon SD. Gastrocnemius-muscle recession (Silfverskiold operation) for spastic equinus deformity in cerebral palsy. J Bone Joint Surg Am 1959;41:1021–8.
5. Nishimoto GS, Attinger CE, Cooper PS. Lengthening the Achilles tendon for the treatment of diabetic plantar forefoot ulceration. Surg Clin North Am 2003;83:707–26.
6. Sammarco GJ, Bagwe MR, Sammarco VJ, et al. The effects of unilateral gastrocsoleus recession. Foot Ankle Int 2006;27:508–11.
7. Myerson MS. Adult acquired flatfoot deformity: treatment of dysfunction of the posterior tibial tendon. Instr Course Lect 1997;46: 393–405.
8. Jeng CL, Bluman EM, Myerson MS. Minimally invasive deltoid ligament reconstruction for stage IV flatfoot deformity. Foot Ankle Int 2011;32:21–30.
9. Deland JT, de Asla RJ, Segal A. Reconstruction of the chronically failed deltoid ligament: a new technique. Foot Ankle Int 2004;25:795–9.
10. Haddad SL, Dedhia S, Ren Y, et al. Deltoid ligament reconstruction: a novel technique with biomechanical analysis. Foot Ankle Int 2010;31:639–51.
11. Dwyer FC. Osteotomy of the calcaneum for pes cavus. J Bone Joint Surg Br 1959;41-B:80–6.
12. Koutsogiannis E. Treatment of mobile flatfoot by displacement osteotomy of the calcaneus. J Bone Joint Surg Br 1971;53:96–100.

13. Fitzgibbons TC. Valgus tilting of the ankle joint after subtalar (hindfoot) fusion: complication or natural progression of valgus hindfoot deformity? Orthopedics 1996; 19:415–23.
14. Resnick RB, Jahss MH, Choueka J, et al. Deltoid ligament forces after tibialis posterior tendon rupture: effects of triple arthrodesis and calcaneal displacement osteotomies. Foot Ankle Int 1995;16:14–20 [Erratum in: Foot Ankle Int 1995;16:314].
15. Wetmore RS, Drennan JC. Long-term results of triple arthrodesis in Charcot-Marie-Tooth disease. J Bone Joint Surg Am 1989;71:417–22.
16. Pell RF 4th, Myerson MS, Schon LC. Clinical outcome after primary triple arthrodesis. J Bone Joint Surg Am 2000;82:47–57.
17. Evans D. Calcaneo-valgus deformity. J Bone Joint Surg Br 1975;57:270–8.
18. Sangeorzan BJ, Mosca V, Hansen ST Jr. Effect of calcaneal lengthening on relationships among the hindfoot, midfoot, and forefoot. Foot Ankle 1993;14:136–41.
19. Haddad SL, Myerson MS, Younger A, et al. SYMPOSIUM: Adult acquired flatfoot deformity. Foot Ankle Int 2011;32:95–111.
20. Cooper PS, Nowak MD, Shaer J. Calcaneocuboid joint pressures with lateral column lengthening (Evans) procedure. Foot Ankle Int 1997;18:199–205.
21. Deland JT, Otis JC, Lee KT, et al. Lateral column lengthening with calcaneocuboid fusion: range of motion in the triple joint complex. Foot Ankle Int 1995;16:729–33.
22. Toolan BC, Sangeorzan BJ, Hansen ST Jr. Complex reconstruction for the treatment of dorsolateral peritalar subluxation of the foot. Early results after distraction arthrodesis of the calcaneocuboid joint in conjunction with stabilization of, and transfer of the flexor digitorum longus tendon to, the midfoot to treat acquired pes planovalgus in adults. J Bone Joint Surg Am 1999;81:1545–60.
23. Cotton F. Foot statistics and surgery. Trans N Engl Surg Soc 1935;18:181–8.
24. Hirose CB, Johnson JE. Plantarflexion opening wedge medial cuneiform osteotomy for correction of fixed forefoot varus associated with flatfoot deformity. Foot Ankle Int 2004;25:568–74.
25. Benthien RA, Parks BG, Guyton GP, et al. Lateral column calcaneal lengthening, flexor digitorum longus transfer, and opening wedge medial cuneiform osteotomy for flexible flatfoot: a biomechanical study. Foot Ankle Int 2007;28:70–7.
26. Mann RA, Beaman DN, Horton GA. Isolated subtalar arthrodesis. Foot Ankle Int 1998;19:511–9.
27. Walker N, Stukenborg C, Savory KM, et al. Hindfoot motion after isolated and combined arthrodesis: measurements in anatomic specimens. Foot Ankle Int 2000; 21:921–7.
28. Graves SC, Mann RA, Graves KO. Triple arthrodesis in older adults. Results after long-term follow-up. J Bone Joint Surg Am 1993;75:355–62.

Update on Stage IV Acquired Adult Flatfoot Disorder

When the Deltoid Ligament Becomes Dysfunctional

Jeremy T. Smith, MD, Eric M. Bluman, MD, PhD*

KEYWORDS

- Posterior tibial tendon dysfunction • Acquired adult flatfoot deformity • Stage IV
- Deltoid ligament • Ankle joint

KEY POINTS

- Stage IV acquired adult flatfoot deformity (AAFD) is present when tibiotalar valgus occurs in association with AAFD.
- Stage IV AAFD can be divided into stage IV-A (flexible deformity without advanced tibiotalar arthritis) and stage IV-B (rigid deformity or flexible deformity with advanced tibiotalar arthritis).
- Stage IV-A can be treated with joint-sparing procedures that include reconstruction of the deltoid ligament.
- Stage IV-B should be treated with a joint-sacrificing procedure.
- Surgical procedures that address stage IV AAFD should be accompanied by procedures to achieve a plantigrade foot.

The posterior tibial tendon plays a central role in maintaining proper foot alignment. Dysfunction of the posterior tibial tendon leads to acquired adult flatfoot deformity (AAFD), a condition that can be both painful and disabling. There are four stages of AAFD, which correlate to increasing deformity. Johnson and Strom[1] described the first three stages in 1989. Stage I AAFD is paratenonitis of the posterior tibial tendon without deformity. The central components of stage II disease are flexible flatfoot deformity with hindfoot valgus, forefoot abduction, and forefoot varus. Stage III is characterized by a fixed hindfoot valgus and often fixed forefoot varus deformity. Myerson[2,3] described a fourth stage, which occurs when the talus tilts into valgus within the ankle mortise secondary to deltoid ligament insufficiency (**Fig. 1**). Stage IV

Department of Orthopaedic Surgery, Brigham Foot and Ankle Center at the Faulkner, Brigham and Women's Hospital, 1153 Centre Street, Suite 56, Boston, MA 02130, USA
* Corresponding author.
E-mail address: ebluman@partners.org

Foot Ankle Clin N Am 17 (2012) 351–360
doi:10.1016/j.fcl.2012.03.011
1083-7515/12/$ – see front matter © 2012 Elsevier Inc. All rights reserved.

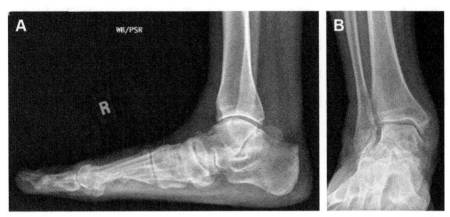

Fig. 1. Stage IV acquired adult flatfoot deformity due to posterior tibial tendon dysfunction. (A) Lateral view of the foot. (B) Anteroposterior view of the ankle with tibiotalar joint valgus angulation.

ankle malalignment is typically accompanied by the deformities present in stages II and III. Stage IV AAFD is subclassified into stage IV-A—flexible ankle valgus without substantial tibiotalar arthritis, and stage IV-B—rigid ankle valgus or flexible ankle valgus with significant tibiotalar arthritis.[4]

ANATOMY AND PATHOGENESIS

The posterior tibialis muscle originates on the posterior tibia, fibula, and interosseous membrane. The posterior tibial tendon (PTT) passes behind the medial malleolus and has a broad insertion at the medial midfoot, a large part of which is on the navicular tuberosity. Additional points of insertion include the sustentaculum tali, cuboid, cuneiforms, and the metatarsal bases of the second, third, and fourth rays. The PTT functions as a powerful inverter of the foot[5] and helps to maintain the foot's longitudinal arch.[6] During normal gait, the PTT pulls the hindfoot into varus, which facilitates locking of the transverse tarsal joint, providing a rigid foot for push-off.

Dysfunction of the posterior tibial tendon has been associated with progressive AAFD.[7] This deformity is thought to relate to the degree and duration of tendon dysfunction. Contributing dynamic deforming factors include the unopposed action of the peroneus brevis (the principal antagonist of the posterior tibialis) and contracture of the triceps surae. The latter exacerbates hindfoot valgus by acting as a hindfoot everter. As hindfoot valgus progresses, the mechanical axis of the leg assumes a medial position relative to the foot with resultant increased tension on soft tissues of the medial ankle. This process leads to progressive failure of the static stabilizers of the medial hindfoot and midfoot, including the spring ligament, plantar fascia, and deltoid ligament complex.[8–12] In cases of advanced AAFD, the spring ligament complex often attenuates or ruptures. Failure of this ligament complex allows the talar head to shift medial and plantar relative to the navicular. As the deltoid ligament complex fails, the talus may assume a valgus position within the ankle mortise.

The deltoid ligament complex consists of superficial and deep components. It serves a critical role in supporting the spring ligament, tibiotalar joint, subtalar joint, and talonavicular joint. The superficial deltoid ligament has been shown to be the primary restraint to tibiotalar valgus angulation.[13–15] Descriptions of the course of the superficial deltoid vary, which may be because of its wide fan-shaped insertion from the navicular to the posterior tibiotalar capsule.[15–19] The tibiocalcaneal ligament is the strongest component of the superficial deltoid.[18] The deep deltoid ligament, originating from the intercollicular groove and posterior colliculus and inserting on the talus, has been shown to principally prevent axial rotation of the talus within the ankle mortise.[13–15]

The deltoid ligament has an important role in preventing valgus deformity of the ankle.

Sequential sectioning of the deltoid ligament complex has demonstrated that both the superficial and deep components prevent tibiotalar tilt. When both components are sectioned, significant valgus talar tilt may occur[17,20,21] and decrease ankle joint contact area by up to 43%.[20]

Chronic deltoid ligament insufficiency can be caused by AAFD,[2,3] trauma, sports-related injuries, triple arthrodesis with valgus malunion,[22] and a poor result after ankle arthroplasty.[23,24] Some data suggest that the deltoid ligament is stressed even after a properly positioned triple arthrodesis.[25,26] Most patients with stage IV AAFD have progressed through stage III disease, although a subset of patients develop valgus talar tilt without a rigid flatfoot deformity, suggesting a possible progression directly from stage II to stage IV AAFD. As described by Bluman and colleagues[4] in 2007, stage IV AAFD may present with or without lateral ankle instability, tibiotalar arthritis, and/or a rigid valgus ankle deformity. Treatment approaches for stage IV AAFD vary depending on the flexibility of the deformity and the degree of ankle arthritis. Stage IV-A is characterized by flexible ankle valgus without significant tibiotalar arthritis. Stage IV-B can be seen with either rigid ankle valgus or flexible ankle valgus with significant tibiotalar arthritis. Patients diagnosed with early stage IV disease may be more likely to have a flexible deformity than those who present later in their disease course.[27]

CLINICAL PRESENTATION AND EVALUATION

Patients with deltoid deficiency and AAFD typically present similarly to patients with stage III AAFD, with the addition of occasional medial-sided ankle pain. Medial-sided pain may have been present earlier in the disease course from PTT paratenonitis. Often this pain will abate after rupture of the PTT and then recur in late-stage disease as the medial ligaments are stressed. Tarsal tunnel neuropathy may also occur with severe valgus deformity.[28,29]

Upon examination, the most likely findings are a pronounced valgus deformity of the hindfoot, an antalgic gait with shortened stride length, and an inability to heel rise. Evaluation should include inspection for abrasions from shoe wear or orthoses. Pain or skin changes beneath the talar head may relate to dorsolateral peritalar subluxation causing prominence at the medial plantar midfoot. Lateral pain may be due to sinus tarsi or subfibular impingement and/or lateral ankle joint arthritis. Other common findings include triceps surae contracture and forefoot varus. Ankle joint range of motion may be severely limited, and care should be taken to accurately measure true ankle dorsiflexion because the fixed hindfoot deformity may falsely elevate perceived ankle dorsiflexion. The ipsilateral knee should also be evaluated because genu valgum can contribute to the foot and ankle deformity.[30]

Proper radiographic evaluation includes imaging both the foot and ankle. Foot radiographs are used to assess for loss of talar head coverage by the navicular (anteroposterior view), dorsolateral peritalar subluxation (anteroposterior and lateral view), increased talo–first metatarsal angle (anteroposterior and lateral views), and decreased calcaneal pitch (lateral view). Weightbearing ankle radiographs will reveal increased talar tilt (anteroposterior and mortise view), the upper limit of which has been reported to be 2°.[31–34] Ankle radiographs are also reviewed to assess tibiotalar arthritis. If talar valgus tilt is present, the flexibility of this deformity must be assessed. Fluoroscopic manipulation is used to evaluate both the flexibility of a valgus deformity and to assess for varus instability, which may be present with concomitant lateral ligament rupture. Comparison contralateral extremity radiographs may be of use.

MANAGEMENT

Some investigators have reported good outcomes with nonsurgical treatment of early-stage AAFD.[35–37] For stage I and II disease, a structured nonoperative protocol with orthoses and physical therapy was shown to have successful subjective and functional outcomes in 83% of patients.[35] For stage III and IV disease, custom molded orthoses such as an Arizona brace may slow the progression of valgus ankle angulation.[36] Yet whereas bracing may control talar tilt, its success in minimizing the development of tibiotalar arthritis is in question. The altered ankle joint biomechanics that accompany deltoid incompetence—decreased joint contact area and increased joint contact forces[20]—may not be adequately corrected with orthoses.

Because of concerns that orthoses do not provide adequate biomechanical correction, some investigators espouse operative treatment of stage IV AAFD in all patients medically fit for surgery.[27,32,38] Severe valgus ankle deformity has historically been treated with tibiotalar fusion. The problem with this approach is that tibiotalar fusion is often accompanied by procedures to correct associated foot deformities such as fusions of the subtalar, talonavicular, calcaneocuboid, and/or midfoot joints. The result of these combined procedures may be a tibiotalocalcaneal or pantalar fusion. Although tibiotalocalcaneal or pantalar fusions are successful in reestablishing a plantigrade foot, many patients report residual pain.[39–41] Objectively, there is increased ambulatory energy expenditure and decreased functionality.[41]

The subclassification of stage IV AAFD into stage IV-A (flexible ankle valgus without significant tibiotalar arthritis) and stage IV-B (rigid ankle valgus or flexible ankle valgus with significant tibiotalar arthritis) has helped to clarify the surgical indications for stage IV AAFD.[4] It is paramount to determine which of these two subclassifications a patient falls into, because stage IV-A is generally treated with ankle joint–sparing procedures and stage IV-B with joint-sacrificing procedures.

Joint-Sparing Operative Management

Joint-sparing operations preserve ankle range of motion, which would otherwise be lost with tibiotalocalcaneal or pantalar fusion. Prior to performing a joint-sparing procedure, the surgeon must understand the deformity. A joint-sparing operation for stage IV AAFD is appropriate for stage IV-A disease. Preoperative or intraoperative fluoroscopic assessment can help to establish the flexibility of the tibiotalar deformity and also identify associated varus instability, if present. If there is associated lateral ligamentous incompetence, an additional lateral ligament reconstruction should be performed. This reconstruction can be accomplished with a variety of techniques, including calcaneofibular ligament imbrication or free gracilis grafting.[42]

Joint-sparing operations rely on reconstruction of the failed deltoid ligament complex. Flatfoot realignment procedures must be also be performed,[43,44] typically prior to medial ligamentous reconstruction in order to facilitate proper tensioning and fixation. The importance of these realignment procedures cannot be overstated, because medial ligament reconstructive attempts will fail if residual coronal plane deformity persists.

Multiple investigators have described techniques for deltoid ligament reconstruction,[45–55] although to date little data exist regarding the outcomes of these various procedures. Ligament reconstruction procedures can be divided into two categories: host-tissue repair operations and graft substitution operations. Although several host-tissue repair procedures have been found to have good short-term results,[50,53] there is concern that chronically injured deltoid ligament tissue may not allow for durable repair over a longer time period.[56] In the absence of long-term data demonstrating the effectiveness of host-tissue repair, several investigators have proposed autograft or allograft tendon reconstructive procedures as an alternative.[27,45,47,54,55] This review focuses on two techniques that have demonstrated reasonable clinical results.[47,48,55]

In 2004, Deland's[47] group published a description of deltoid ligament reconstruction using peroneus longus tendon autograft in patients with stage IV flatfoot.[47] In this procedure, the peroneus longus tendon is transected proximally and then passed through a tunnel in the talus from lateral to medial. The tendon is then passed from medial to lateral through a tunnel in the medial malleolus to replicate the fibers of the deep deltoid. Fixation is achieved either by suturing to a screw at the fibula or by stapling at the lateral tibia. In a study of 5 patients with a minimum 2-year follow-up, average correction of valgus talar tilt was from 10° preoperative valgus to 4° postoperative valgus.[47] A follow-up publication examining the same five patients at a mean 8.9 years postoperatively reported a mean valgus talar tilt of 2°, mean Foot and Ankle Orthopaedic Surgery score of 68 (maximum, 100), mean SF-36v2 score of 76 (maximum,100), mean visual analogue scale of 4 (maximum, 10), and mean ankle range of motion of 47°.[48] A criticism of this procedure is that it fails to reconstruct the superficial component of the deltoid ligament complex, which has been shown to be the primary restraint to valgus ankle angulation.[13–15] Furthermore, there is concern about donor-site morbidity from the use of autograft tendon, and the senior author of this technique now reportedly uses Achilles tendon allograft instead of peroneal tendon autograft.[48]

In 2011, Jeng and colleagues[55] reported the outcomes of a minimally invasive deltoid ligament reconstruction for stage IV-A flatfoot deformity (**Fig. 2**). This technique, described initially in 2007,[27] uses hamstring allograft tendon to reconstruct both the deep and superficial components of the deltoid ligament complex. A 20-cm graft is split longitudinally to create two limbs, leaving 6 cm intact as a single limb. The single limb is passed through a tibial tunnel parallel to the ankle joint surface at the distal tibial physeal scar and fixed using a bioabsorbable PLLA interference screw. The graft is subcutaneously passed distally and one limb is secured by interference screw through a talar tunnel to recreate the deep deltoid fibers. The remaining limb is then passed through a calcaneal tunnel and fixed with an interference screw to recreate the superficial deltoid (**Fig. 3**).

Candidates for this minimally invasive deltoid ligament reconstruction had (1) ankle pain refractory to nonsurgical care, (2) rigid hindfoot valgus and forefoot abduction deformity consistent with stage IV AAFD, (3) valgus talar tilt of at least 3° that was (4) passively correctable tibiotalar valgus documented fluoroscopically and had (5) at least 2 mm of lateral tibiotalar cartilage remaining.[55] At an average of 36 months postoperatively, 5 of 8 patients were deemed to have had a successful outcome with a correction to less than 3° of valgus talar tilt, preserved lateral tibiotalar joint space, SF-12 functional scores equivalent to age-matched normative scores, and mean ankle range of motion of 42°. Patients with a preoperative valgus talar tilt of greater than 10° had inferior outcomes. The investigators concluded that this procedure is appropriate for a carefully selected population with stage IV-A AAFD.

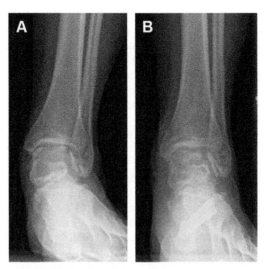

Fig. 2. Stage IV-A acquired adult flatfoot deformity reconstruction using a minimally invasive deltoid ligament reconstruction. (*A*) Preoperative anteroposterior view of the ankle showing a valgus deformity of the tibiotalar joint. (*B*) Postoperative anteroposterior view showing correction of the deformity.

Another technique that shows early promise in biomechanical studies was described by Haddad and colleagues[54] in 2010. This reconstruction attempts to anatomically recreate both limbs of the deltoid ligament complex using a looped semitendinosis allograft passed through a drill hole at the intercollicular groove of the medial malleolus to the anterior distal tibia.[54] One end of the tendon is then secured to the talus through a tunnel to recreate the deep tibiotalar limb whereas the other is secured to the calcaneus to recreate the superficial tibiocalcaneal limb. A cadaveric biomechanical analysis showed no statistical difference in angular displacement under load between reconstructed ankles and cadaveric ankles with an intact native deltoid ligament. The conclusions from this cadaveric study were that this technique restores eversion and external rotation stability to the talus under low torque. The investigators themselves mention one of the biggest concerns with this technique, which is that to date there are no published clinical outcomes. Although the biomechanical data are promising, in vivo healing and durability are not yet known.

Joint-Sacrificing Operative Management

Patients with rigid valgus talar tilt or severe tibiotalar arthritis are not appropriate for an ankle joint–sparing procedure, but rather should be considered candidates for either a tibiotalocalcaneal or pantalar arthrodesis.[4,27] These procedures are reliable but are not without potential problems because many patients have residual pain, nonunion, increased ambulatory energy expenditure, and decreased functionality.[39–41] An alternative approach to stage IV-B AAFD is to realign the weightbearing axis with a hindfoot fusion and then perform a total ankle arthroplasty.[38,57,58] Although this approach is an attractive option, persistent valgus malalignment has been reported in 50% of patients after this combination of procedures.[58] Another option for a stage IV-B AAFD is a combined total ankle arthroplasty and deltoid ligament reconstruction. Although little has been published on this topic, the

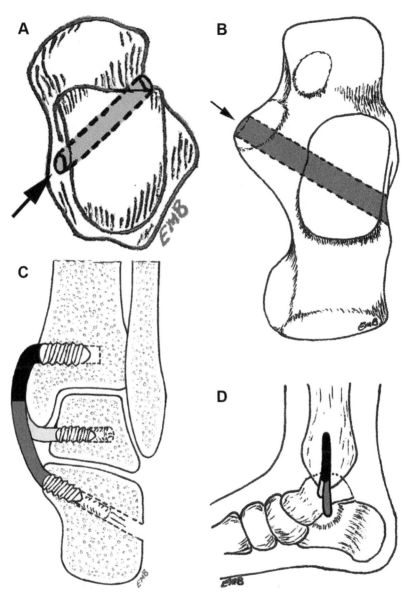

Fig. 3. Minimally invasive deltoid ligament reconstruction. Disarticulated superior view of the talus (*A*) and calcaneus (*B*) demonstrating the trajectory of graft limbs with arrows marking the entry site of the graft in the bones. (*C*) Coronal sectional view showing how graft limbs are anchored. (*D*) Medial view of the ankle showing tibial (*black*), talar (*light gray*), and calcaneal (*dark gray*) limbs of graft.

minimally invasive ligament reconstruction technique described by Jeng and colleagues[55] would be a good choice because of the small incision and avoidance of large skin bridges. Proper implant selection is critical, because a large tibial keel will interfere with proper graft tunnel placement.

SUMMARY

Deltoid ligament complex insufficiency is a fundamental pathologic component of stage IV AAFD. Failure of the deltoid ligament allows the talus to tilt into valgus within the ankle mortise. If left untreated, ankle joint biomechanics are altered and may lead to debilitating tibiotalar arthritis. All surgical treatments that address the valgus talar tilt seen with stage IV AAFD require accompanying procedures to properly realign the hindfoot. Stage IV AAFD can be subdivided into two groups. Patients with a flexible ankle deformity without advanced tibiotalar arthritis (stage IV-A) can be considered for a joint-sparing procedure. A variety of procedures have been described, but long-term follow-up studies have yet to determine which of these techniques is optimal. Patients with a rigid valgus ankle deformity or a flexible deformity accompanied by advanced tibiotalar arthritis (stage IV-B) should be considered for a joint-sacrificing procedure. To date, the most reliable results for stage IV-B AAFD have been reported with either tibiotalocalcaneal or pan-talar arthrodesis.

REFERENCES

1. Johnson KA, Strom DE. Tibialis posterior tendon dysfunction. Clin Orthop 1989;(239): 196–206.
2. Myerson MS. Adult acquired flatfoot deformity; treatment of dysfunction of the posterior tibial tendon. Inst Course Lect 1997;46:393–405.
3. Myerson MS. Adult acquired flatfoot deformity. Treatment of dysfunction of the posterior tibial tendon. J Bone Joint Surg Am 1996;78:780–92.
4. Bluman EM, Title CI, Myerson MS. Posterior tibial tendon rupture: a refined classification system. Foot Ankle Clin 2007;12:233–49.
5. Mann R, Inman VT. Phasic activity of intrinsic muscles of the foot. J Bone Joint Surg Am 1964;46:469–81.
6. Kitoaka HB, Luo ZP, An KN. Effect of the posterior tibial tendon on the arch of the foot during simulated weightbearing: biomechanical analysis. Foot Ankle Int 1997;18(1): 43–6.
7. Mann RA, Thompson FM. Rupture of the posterior tibial tendon causing flat foot: surgical treatment. J Bone Joint Surg Am 1985;67:556–61.
8. Deland JT. The acquired flatfoot and spring ligament complex. Foot Ankle Clin 2001;6:129–35.
9. Deland JT, de Asla RJ, Sung IH, et al. Posterior tibial tendon insufficiency: which ligaments are involved? Foot Ankle Int 2005;26(6):427–35.
10. Balen PF, Helms CA. Association of posterior tibial tendon injury with spring ligament injury, sinus tarsi abnormality, and plantar fasciitis on MR imaging. AJR Am J Roentgenol 2001;176(5):1137–43.
11. Yao L, Gentili A, Cracchiolo A. MR imaging findings in spring ligament insufficiency. Skeletal Radiol 1999;28(5):245–50.
12. Gazdag AR, Cracchiolo A 3rd. Rupture of the posterior tibial tendon. Evaluation of injury of the spring ligament and clinical assessment of tendon transfer and ligament repair. J Bone Joint Surg Am 1997;79(5):675–81.
13. Rasmussen O. Stability of the ankle joint. Analysis of the function and traumatology of the ankle ligaments. Acta Orthop Scand Suppl 1985;211:1–75.
14. Rasmussen O, Kromann-Andersen C. Experimental ankle injuries. Analysis of the traumatology of the ankle ligaments. Acta Orthop Scand 1983;54:356–62.
15. Rasmussen O, Kromann-Andersen C, Boe S. Deltoid ligament. Functional analysis of the medial collateral ligamentous apparatus of the ankle joint. Acta Orthop Scand 1983;54:36–44.

16. Boss AP, Hintermann B. Anatomical study of the medial ankle ligament complex. Foot Ankle Int. 2002;23:547–53.
17. Harper MC. Deltoid ligament: an anatomical evaluation of function. Foot Ankle 1987;8:19–22.
18. Pankovich AM, Shivaram MS. Anatomical basis of variability in injuries of the medial malleolus and the deltoid ligament. I. Anatomical studies. Acta Orthop Scand 1979; 50:217–23.
19. Siegler S, Block J, Schneck CD. The mechanical characteristics of the collateral ligaments of the human ankle joint. Foot Ankle 1988;8:234–42.
20. Earll M, Wayne J, Brodrick C, et al. Contribution of the deltoid ligament to ankle joint contact characteristics: a cadaver study. Foot Ankle Int 1996;17(6):317–24.
21. Close JR. Some applications of the functional anatomy of the ankle joint. J Bone Joint Surg Am 1956;38:761–81.
22. Haddad SL, Myerson MS, Pell RF, et al. Clinical and radiographic outcome of revision surgery for failed triple arthrodesis. Foot Ankle Int 1997;18(8):489–99.
23. Haskell A, Mann RA. Ankle arthroplasty with preoperative coronal plane deformity: short-term results. Clin Orthop 2004;424:98–103.
24. Stamatis ED, Myerson MS. How to avoid specific complications of total ankle replacement. Foot Ankle Clin 2002;7(4):178–84.
25. Song S, Lee S, O'Malley M, et al. Deltoid ligament strain after correction of acquired flatfoot deformity by triple arthrodesis. Foot Ankle Int 2000;21(7):573–7.
26. Resnick RB, Jahss MH, Choueka J, et al. Deltoid ligament forces after tibialis posterior tendon rupture: effects of triple arthrodesis and calcaneal displacement osteotomies. Foot Ankle Int 1995;16(1):14–20.
27. Bluman EM, Myerson M. Stage IV posterior tibial tendon rupture. Foot Ankle Clin 2007;12(2):341–62.
28. Francis H, March L, Terenty T, et al. Benign joint hypermobility with neuropathy: documentation and mechanism of tarsal tunnel syndrome. J Rheumatol 1987;14(3): 577–81.
29. Daniels TR, Lau JT, Hearn TC. The effects of foot position and load on tibial nerve tension. Foot Ankle Int 1988;19(2):73–8.
30. Sobel M, Stern S, Manoli A. The association of posterior tibialis tendon insufficiency with valgus osteoarthritis of the knee. Am J Knee Surg 1992;5:59.
31. Michelson JD, Helgemo SL Jr. Kinematics of the axially loaded ankle. Foot Ankle Int 1995;16(9):577–82.
32. Kelly IP, Nunley JA. Treatment of stage 4 adult acquired flatfoot. Foot Ankle Clin 2001;6(1):167–78.
33. Karlsson J, Bergsten T, Lansinger O, et al. Surgical treatment of chronic lateral instability of the ankle. A new procedure. Am J Sports Med 1989;17(2):268–73.
34. Karlsson J, Bergsten T, Lansinger O, et al. Reconstruction of the lateral ligaments of the ankle for chronic lateral instability. J Bone Joint Surg Am 1988;70(4):581–8.
35. Alvarez RG, Marini A, Schmitt C, et al. Stage I and II posterior tibial tendon dysfunction treated by a structured nonoperative management protocol: an orthosis and exercise program. Foot Ankle Int 2006;27(1):2–8.
36. Wapner KL, Chao W. Nonoperative treatment of posterior tibial tendon dysfunction. Clin Orthop 1999;365:39–45.
37. Chao W, Wapner KL, Lee TH, et al. Non-operative treatment of posterior tibial tendon dysfunction. Foot Ankle Int 1996;17:736–41.
38. Bohay DR, Anderson JG. Stage IV posterior tibial tendon insufficiency: the tilted ankle. Foot Ankle Clin 2003;8(3):619–36.

39. Barrett GR, Meyer LC, Bray EW 3rd, et al. Pantalar arthrodesis: a long-term follow-up. Foot Ankle 1981;1(5):279–83.
40. Chou LB, Mann RA, Yaszay B, et al. Tibiotalocalcaneal arthrodesis. Foot Ankle Int 2000;21(10):804–8.
41. Papa JA, Myerson MS. Pantalar and tibiotalocalcaneal arthrodesis for post-traumatic osteoarthrosis of the ankle and hindfoot. J Bone Joint Surg Am 1992;74(7):1042–9.
42. Coughlin MJ, Schenck RC Jr, Grebing BR, et al. Comprehensive reconstruction of the lateral ankle for chronic instability using a free gracilis graft. Foot Ankle Int 2004;25(4):231–41.
43. Haddad SL, Myerson MS, Younger A, et al. Adult acquired flatfoot deformity. Foot Ankle Int 2011;32(1):95–111.
44. Anderson R, Davis W. Management of the adult flatfoot deformity. In: Myerson MS, editor. Foot and ankle disorders. 1st edition. Philadelphia (PA): WB Saunders and Co; 2000. p. 1017–39.
45. Kitoaka HB, Luo ZP, An KN. Reconstruction operations for acquired flatfoot: biomechanical evaluation. Foot Ankle Int 1998;19(4):203–7.
46. Goldner JL, Keats PK, Bassett FH 3rd, et al. Progressive talipes equinovalgus due to trauma or degeneration of the posterior tibial tendon and medial plantar ligaments. Orthop Clin North Am 1974;5(1):39–51.
47. Deland JT, de Asla RJ, Segal A. Reconstruction of the chronically failed deltoid ligament: a new technique. Foot Ankle Int 2004;25(11):795–9.
48. Ellis SJ, Williams BR, Wagshul AD, et al. Deltoid ligament reconstruction with peroneus longus autograft in flatfoot deformity. Foot Ankle Int 2010;31(9):781–9.
49. Boyer MI, Bowen V, Weiler P. Reconstruction of a severe grinding injury to the medial malleolus and the deltoid ligament of the ankle using a free plantaris tendon graft and vascularized gracilis free muscle transfer: a case report. J Trauma 1994;36(3):454–7.
50. Raikin SM, Myerson MS. Surgical repair of ankle injuries to the deltoid ligament. Foot Ankle Clin 1999;4(4):745–53.
51. Kelikian K, Kelikian A. Disruptions of the deltoid ligament. In: Disorders of the ankle. 1st edition. Philadelphia: WB Saunders; 1985. p. 339–70.
52. McCormack AP, Ching RP, Sangeorzan BJ. Biomechanics of procedures used in adult flatfoot deformity. Foot Ankle Clin 2001;6(1):15.–23, v.
53. Hintermann B, Valderrabano V, Boss A, et al. Medial ankle instability: an exploratory, prospective study of fifty-two cases. Am J Sports Med 2004;32(1):183–90.
54. Haddad SL, Dedhia S, Ren Y, et al. Deltoid ligament reconstruction: a novel technique with biomechanical analysis. Foot Ankle Int 2010;31(7):639–51.
55. Jeng CL, Bluman EM, Myerson MS. Minimally invasive deltoid ligament reconstruction for stage IV flatfoot deformity. Foot Ankle Int 2011;32(1):21–30.
56. Hurschler C, Provenzano PP, Vanderby R Jr. Scanning electron microscopic characterization of healing and normal rat ligament microstructure under slack and loaded conditions. Connect Tissue Res 2003;44(2):59–68.
57. Walling AK. Chapter 19: stage IV flatfoot: alternatives to tibiocalcaneal or pantalar procedures. In: Nunley JA, Pfeffer GB, Sanders R, et al, editors. Advanced reconstruction of the foot and ankle. Rosemont (IL): American Academy of Orthopaedic Surgeons; 2004. p. 123–6.
58. Hall C, Agel J, Hansen S, et al. Complications in the treatment of stage IV adult-acquired flatfoot. Presented at the American Orthopaedic Foot and Ankle 22nd Summer Meeting. La Jolla (CA), July 14-16, 2006.

Index

Note: Page numbers of article titles are in **boldface** type.

Foot Ankle Clin N Am 17 (2012) 361–387
http://dx.doi.org/10.1016/S1083-7515(12)00037-X
1083-7515/12/$ – see front matter © 2012 Elsevier Inc. All rights reserved.

foot.theclinics.com

Moving?

Make sure your subscription moves with you!

To notify us of your new address, find your **Clinics Account Number** (located on your mailing label above your name), and contact customer service at:

Email: journalscustomerservice-usa@elsevier.com

800-654-2452 (subscribers in the U.S. & Canada)
314-447-8871 (subscribers outside of the U.S. & Canada)

Fax number: 314-447-8029

Elsevier Health Sciences Division
Subscription Customer Service
3251 Riverport Lane
Maryland Heights, MO 63043

*To ensure uninterrupted delivery of your subscription, please notify us at least 4 weeks in advance of move.

Printed and bound by CPI Group (UK) Ltd, Croydon, CR0 4YY

03/10/2024

01040445-0003